The Big Back Book

Tips and Tricks for Therapists

Jane Johnson, MSc
Chartered Physiotherapist
Health and Care Professions Council
Chartered Society of Physiotherapy
United Kingdom

907 illustrations

Thieme
Stuttgart • New York • Delhi • Rio de Janeiro

Library of Congress Cataloging-in-Publication Data is available from the publisher.

Section opener images: Reproduced with permission from Gilroy & MacPherson, Atlas of Anatomy, 3rd edition, © 2016, Thieme Publishers, New York, New York. Illustrators: Markus Voll and Karl Wesker.

© 2017 by Georg Thieme Verlag KG

Thieme Publishers Stuttgart
Rüdigerstrasse 14, 70469 Stuttgart, Germany
+49 [0]711 8931 421, customerservice@thieme.de

Thieme Publishers New York
333 Seventh Avenue, New York, NY 10001 USA
+1 800 782 3488, customerservice@thieme.com

Thieme Publishers Delhi
A-12, Second Floor, Sector-2, Noida-201301
Uttar Pradesh, India
+91 120 45 566 00, customerservice@thieme.in

Thieme Publishers Rio, Thieme Publicações Ltda.
Edifício Rodolpho de Paoli, 25º andar
Av. Nilo Peçanha, 50 – Sala 2508
Rio de Janeiro 20020-906, Brasil
+55 21 3172 2297 / +55 21 3172 1896

Cover design: Thieme Publishing Group
Typesetting by Thomson Digital, India

Printed in Italy by LEGO S.p.A   5 4 3 2 1

ISBN 978-3-13-204821-8

Also available as an e-book:
eISBN 978-3-13-204831-7

Important note: Medicine is an ever-changing science undergoing continual development. Research and clinical experience are continually expanding our knowledge, in particular our knowledge of proper treatment and drug therapy. Insofar as this book mentions any dosage or application, readers may rest assured that the authors, editors, and publishers have made every effort to ensure that such references are in accordance with **the state of knowledge at the time of production of the book.**

Nevertheless, this does not involve, imply, or express any guarantee or responsibility on the part of the publishers in respect to any dosage instructions and forms of applications stated in the book. **Every user is requested to examine carefully** the manufacturers' leaflets accompanying each drug and to check, if necessary in consultation with a physician or specialist, whether the dosage schedules mentioned therein or the contraindications stated by the manufacturers differ from the statements made in the present book. Such examination is particularly important with drugs that are either rarely used or have been newly released on the market. Every dosage schedule or every form of application used is entirely at the user's own risk and responsibility. The authors and publishers request every user to report to the publishers any discrepancies or inaccuracies noticed. If errors in this work are found after publication, errata will be posted at www.thieme.com on the product description page.

Some of the product names, patents, and registered designs referred to in this book are in fact registered trademarks or proprietary names even though specific reference to this fact is not always made in the text. Therefore, the appearance of a name without designation as proprietary is not to be construed as a representation by the publisher that it is in the public domain.

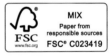

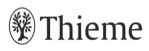

To all of the students and fellow therapists whose comments over the years have contributed to my knowledge of assessment and treatment techniques. Also, to the patients from whom honest feedback has proved invaluable.

Contents

Preface

This book came about following the delivery, over many years, of a series of workshops on the specific topics of neck and back assessment and treatment. The workshops focused on a simple premise: to share tips that I had picked up over many years working as a physical therapist and massage therapist. The workshops tended to attract therapists who lacked confidence or who felt that they had not received comprehensive training in the area of assessment and treatment, yet who themselves attracted patients for whom such treatment was required. The workshops also attracted therapists who were frustrated at not achieving what they felt were good results for their clients and who thirsted to seek answers regarding different techniques. Perhaps it was because some of the therapists in attendance felt they lacked knowledge, or because some were motivated to vary their approach, that these workshops generated much discussion and debate, and sharing of ideas. I began keeping notes for the purposes of introducing new ideas into the workshops and generating further discussion. I formed the idea for writing three separate books containing tips and tricks for therapists: *The Neck, The Thorax, and The Lumbar Spine*.

During the workshops, participants were invited to give and receive different assessment and treatment techniques, the facilitation of which hugely informed my own practice. This is the reason why the book is partly dedicated to those participants. Many times over the course of delivering the workshops, I was asked questions to which I had no answer, and this fired my own enthusiasm for investigation. The more questions I was asked, and the more I experimented, the less I felt I knew. I continued to keep copious notes. What was apparent was that the participating therapists each had different and often contrasting responses to which techniques they preferred and found helpful. This is why you will discover that suggestions throughout *The Big Back Book* are just that—suggestions. I have deliberately avoided being prescriptive with regard to methods of assessment and treatment.

Although I had made a tentative foray into self-publishing and produced *The Neck* and *The Thorax*, I was delighted when Thieme Medical Publishers agreed to buy these titles from me and to combine them with *The Lumbar Spine* to create the book you have here.

I continue to feel that there is much to learn myself about these topics. Nevertheless, this book is based on the questions I was able to answer during those workshops and is offered to you as a collection of examples of those methods that have worked well for me over the years. It is a book I wish I had had early on in my career.

Jane Johnson

Acknowledgments

I would like to thank Lee Lawrence for formatting my manuscript and illustrations and for massive contribution to the images in this book, for addressing many editorial amendments, and for liaising with the publishers on my behalf regarding technical elements of the book.

Thank you Jair Herculano for producing numerous line drawings so quickly and on schedule.

I would also like to thank Angelika Findgott of Thieme Medical Publishers for her immediate enthusiastic response to this book, and to the team at Thieme for believing, like me, that therapists will benefit from the dissemination of this information.

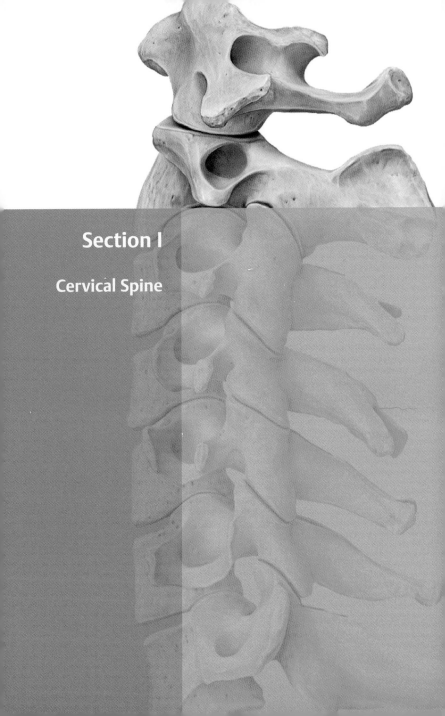

Section I

Cervical Spine

Introduction

The neck is the part of the body that many therapists admit they are sometimes scared to treat. It is crammed with nerves, and we are rightfully taught to take care when working on this region of the spine, but to such an extent that some therapists become anxious about treating it with anything other than very general, gentle massage.

Of course, gentle massage involving effleurage and petrissage is all that is sometimes required. But often the relief provided is short term; the client's problem persists or you feel "stuck" as to what advice you can give your client to help them self-manage their problem. This section provides you with ideas for the assessment, treatment, and aftercare of those clients who come to you complaining of problems such as general neck pain or stiffness—the kind of clients so many of us come across on a regular basis.

If you have ever felt uncertain about how to treat this part of the body, and your skills and confidence need a boost, then this section of the book is for you.

The tips and tricks provided here are effective and safe. They fall within the remit of qualified therapists. If you are a newly qualified therapist or have not practiced for some time, the information you find here will improve your understanding and help you gain confidence. If you are an experienced therapist, I hope you too will find something useful among these tips.

It is assumed that you have consulted your client, taken a general medical history, and decided that your client is safe to be assessed and treated, and that they have given consent for this.

Each of the three chapters in this section contains a list of tips. Within these, embedded within the text, you will find additional tips. You will also find common questions boxed.

Chapter I

Neck Assessment

Chapter 1 Neck Assessment

In this chapter you will find lots of *tips* on how to assess someone who comes to you with a neck complaint. This might be something as simple as a stiff neck, a sore neck, feeling tense after sitting for long periods of time at work, or perhaps even an odd "niggle" in the neck caused by an injury that happened many years ago. It could be someone you have been treating for many months or a new client.

The *tips and tricks* you will find here are not arranged in any particular order. The information here is not designed to replace any training you have had. Instead, it is designed to support and enhance your existing skills and is crammed with the kinds of *tips* you may not have come across, *tips and tricks* I have picked up over the years, and

which I hope you too will find beneficial in your practice. Of course, there will be material with which you are familiar, but I am hoping that you will discover a selection of assessment tips which make you think, "Ah, I haven't tried that, maybe that will work!"

Most therapists reading this book will be sensible enough to know that you would not carry out any of these assessments on a person with an acute injury to their neck, such as whiplash. You will find only a few *cautions* written into the text in this chapter, and the reason is that the majority of these assessments are perfectly safe for the majority of people you are likely to be assessing. Where *special caution* is needed, this has been stated, so please read the whole tip before attempting the assessment.

Tip 1: Assessing Range of Movement

When a client comes to you with a neck problem, one of the simplest assessments you can make—once you have finished asking questions—is to observe which movements they can (and cannot) perform with their neck. You may already be doing this and may know that this is called a range of movement (ROM) test. Because you are going to ask the client to perform the movements themselves, this is an *active* ROM test. You may have heard of passive ROM tests, where the therapist takes a joint through its ROM, but in this section, for this part of the body, we are only going to do active ROM tests.

The neck can move in six ranges for the purposes of this assessment: flexion/extension, right lateral flexion/left lateral flexion, and right rotation/left rotation.

A good place to start when assessing the neck is to demonstrate to your client what it is you want them to do, and then to watch how they perform the movements and to note what they say.

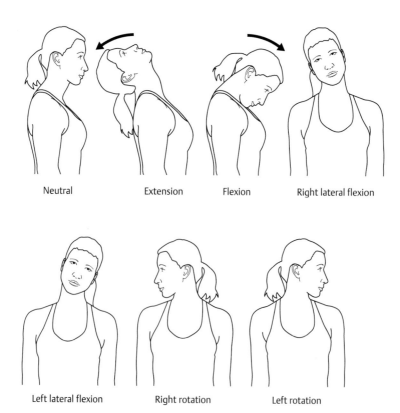

Neutral   Extension   Flexion   Right lateral flexion

Left lateral flexion   Right rotation   Left rotation

Question: Does it matter which movement the client performs first?

No. If you are new to this form of assessment, one tip is always to perform the movements in the same order, with every client. For example, flexion, then extension and back to neutral; right rotation, then left rotation and back to neutral; right lateral flexion, then left lateral flexion and back to neutral. That way, you are unlikely to miss anything. However, there may be times when you need to make an exception. For example, if a client has already told you that they experience discomfort on a particular movement—rotation of their head to the right, for example—it is sometimes a good idea to ask them to perform this particular movement *last*. The reason for this is that if the client experiences discomfort at the start of the assessment, they may be less willing to continue and you may not discover which movements they can and cannot make. So, if a client tells you that they experience discomfort on looking over their right shoulder when trying to reverse their car, make right rotation the last ROM that you test, checking the other five movements first.

TIP: Make sure that your client does not move their shoulders when performing ROM tests. Clients with neck pain or a stiff neck have a tendency to twist at the waist and move their thorax in order to rotate to the right or to the left, instead of rotating their neck. Similarly, when asked to perform lateral flexion, they have a tendency to raise their shoulders: if lateral flexion to the right is uncomfortable or difficult, they raise their left shoulder, thus appearing to be able to move in this direction when in fact the movement is generated from their torso. Check for these "cheating" movements by paying close attention to your client's shoulders during the test. If you see movement in the shoulders, instruct your client to start again, while keeping their shoulders stationary. By asking the client to keep their shoulders stationary, the limitations in their cervical ROM become more apparent and you therefore get a more accurate picture of what they can and cannot do with their neck.

Question: Does it matter where you stand when carrying out this assessment?

Some therapists stand behind their clients when assessing active cervical ROM. The advantage is that the therapist can observe the cervical spine. The disadvantage is that the client may feel anxious having someone stand behind them, even though the cervical ROM test is quick to perform: as you know, people are protective of their necks, more so if they are in pain or have suffered neck problems in the past. Standing in front of your client, you have the advantage of being able to observe their facial expressions. This position is also more conducive to the development of rapport.

Question: Are active ROM tests safe for all clients?

Active ROM tests are safe for most people because everyone moves their head through these ranges—and combinations of these ranges—during the day. Active ROM tests may *not* be safe in certain, very specific, circumstances: following an accident or following surgery to the neck, for example. This section is not designed to help you assess people with cervical trauma. Also, there may be a small group of people for whom caution is needed when asking them to perform active movements involving the head and the neck. For example, active ROM tests should be performed with caution if, when taking the client's medical history, you discover your subject suffers from an inner ear disorder such as Ménière's disease. Another example is if they report experiencing dizziness when they look up to the ceiling.

Question: When caution is needed, what instructions might you give the client prior to them performing the test?

Instruct them to move their head *slowly* or to stop if they feel in any way dizzy or unwell.

Tip 2: How to Tell What Is a "Normal" Range of Movement

So you have tested your client's active cervical ROM. As they were performing the movements you found yourself asking, "How do I know what is a 'normal' ROM in the neck?" Well, there are many books in which normal ranges of movement can be found. One such book is *The Clinical Measurement of Joint Motion* by the American Academy of Orthopaedic Surgeons (Green and Heckman 1994). This has clear illustrations and focuses only on this topic, so it is easy to follow.

However, a good *tip* is simply to assess a lot of people. By doing this you will soon get to build up a kind of visual database, a set of images in your mind as to what is normal and what is not. When you see someone who can only flex their head to the side a little, you will know that they have a ROM *less than* the norm. Conversely, when a client effortlessly bends their head to the side so that their ear appears to almost touch their shoulder, you will know that they have a ROM *greater* than the norm.

Normal Range of Movement		
Range of movement	**Neutral position**	**Example**
Flexion This could be measured in 0–90 degrees from the neutral position. Norm = about 38 degrees Or, it could be measured crudely in terms of how many centimeters (or inches) the subject's chin is from their sternum.		This person has about 45 degrees of flexion. Their chin is less than 1 cm from their sternum. They would appear to have a greater degree of cervical flexion than most people.
Extension This could be measured in 0–90 degrees from the neutral position. Norm = about 38 degrees Or, it could be measured crudely in terms of how many centimeters (or inches) the subject's chin is from their sternum.		This person has about 30 degrees of extension. Their chin is about 22.5 cm from their chest. This appears to be slightly less than a normal range.
Lateral flexion This could be measured in 0–90 degrees from the neutral position. Norm = about 43 degrees Or, you could measure crudely how far the client's ear is from their shoulder.		In this example, our subject has about 22 degrees of left lateral flexion, less than the norm.
Rotation This could be measured in 0–90 degrees from the neutral position. Norm = about 45 degrees		

Use the table on the opposite page to help you record five neck assessments. The illustrations at the top of the table are a reminder of the six movements you need to check. One assessment has been filled in for you, for a subject called Mrs. Brown, aged 64. From the table you can see that she has 30 degrees of flexion and 20 degrees of extension; 30 degrees of right rotation and 25 degrees of left rotation; and 10 degrees of right lateral flexion and 20 degrees of left lateral flexion.

TIP: Assess 10 people who drive for a living or who do a *lot* of driving; 10 people who are older than 70 years; 10 people who have sustained a whiplash injury in the past 5 years (providing they are safe to be assessed now, of course); 10 people who maintain a static posture for long periods of time; and 10 people who regularly perform yoga. These are arbitrary selections, but you get the idea. By assessing similar groups of people, you will soon discover interesting similarities among clients. For example, if you have not done so already, you may discover that, as we age, the range through which we can actively move our neck decreases. Also, movement decreases in one or more ranges following injury if the client has not been properly rehabilitated; and people who regularly perform yoga may have an increase in cervical range, or may maintain their cervical range for longer as they age.

Subject	Flexion	Extension	Right rotation	Left rotation	Right lateral flexion	Left lateral flexion
Mrs. Brown aged 64	30	20	30	25	10	20

It would be wrong to say that all elderly people have a reduced ROM in their neck. Some may have an increase in range—maybe they are fitness enthusiasts and include neck stretches in their routines, or perhaps they had increased mobility to start with. You get the idea. So, while we do not want to pigeonhole people, the more people you assess, the more likely you are to be able to identify when a client has a ROM that is greater or less than normal, taking into account their age, occupation, lifestyle, and health factors.

The problem with measuring ROM is that people's necks can "hinge" in different places. That is, some of the vertebrae can remain "stuck," while others move more freely, so the movement we observe is not coming equally from each of the seven cervical vertebrae. Vertebrae do not form hinge joints, as you know, but the movement impairment that is sometimes observed when people perform ROM assessments may be thought of as a hinging *movement*.

Question: What if a client reports a problem involving movement, yet when you test them, they appear to have a normal ROM? That is, flexion, extension, lateral flexion (both left and right), and rotation (both left and right) all appear fine, with little or minimal discomfort.

There are many factors contributing to neck discomfort (movement is *one* of them). The thing to remember is that in daily life we *combine* these movements. For example, if you are holding this text slightly lower than horizontal in order to read it, your neck may be a little flexed. If you were to keep your neck flexed but look over your right shoulder, you are now combining forward flexion with right rotation. Similarly, if you look up into the sky and trace the path of an aircraft as it passes overhead, your neck is in extension and will involve a degree of rotation, depending on which way the aircraft is moving. Try rubbing your left ear on your left shoulder by moving your head. You are now combining left lateral flexion with both right and left rotation. So, it may be that a client's condition is aggravated not by one movement, but by a combination of movements, and this is worth remembering as it provides further clues that will help you determine what the problem, and the appropriate treatment, might be.

Tip 3: Using a Goniometer to Measure Cervical ROM

If you want to be more accurate in your cervical ROM measurement, you could use a goniometer. Begin with your client seated, preferably with their back supported and feet flat on the floor. Then, position your goniometer as shown in this tip and measure the different ranges. Follow the instructions provided on the following pages to help you to measure flexion, extension, lateral flexion, and rotation.

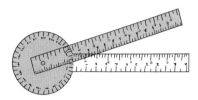

Questions to ask yourself:

How easy did I find using a goniometer to measure cervical ROM?

Did I find any particular aspects easier than others? For example, was it easier for me to measure rotation than lateral flexion?

What could I do differently next time to improve my skill in using a goniometer to measure cervical ROM?

Would using a larger or smaller goniometer help?

Was the client positioned correctly? Could I change the position in any way to make measuring easier or more accurate?

How good was I at giving instructions to my subject? Did they understand? Is there anything I need to do differently next time?

How easy was it for me to record my findings?

Questions to ask about your client:

How do their ROM measurements compare with other subjects of their age and gender?

Are there differences in left- and right-sided readings?

Have these measurements changed over time and if so, in what way?

In what way might a ROM finding relate to my client's daily life—does decreased (or increased) ROM make any daily tasks more difficult?

Would helping to alter ROM improve my client's quality of life in any way? For example, if they had greater cervical rotation, would that help when they are looking over their shoulder to reverse their car?

How might I explain ROM findings to my client in a way that is reassuring?

Measuring Neck Flexion with a Goniometer

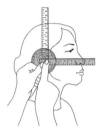

1. Position the center of your goniometer over the external auditory meatus.

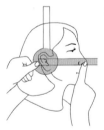

2. Ensure that the arm of the goniometer that is to be stationary is perpendicular to the floor.

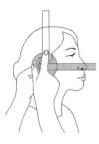

3. Align the arm of the goniometer that is to move with nares.

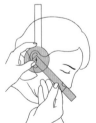

4. Ask your client to take their chin as close to their chest as possible and, as they do this, move the arm of the goniometer to keep it aligned with nares. Be sure to keep the stationary arm of the goniometer fixed. Take your measurement.

Measuring Neck Extension with a Goniometer

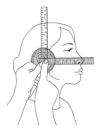

1. Position the center of your goniometer over the external auditory meatus.

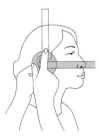

2. Ensure that the arm of the goniometer that is to be stationary is perpendicular to the floor.

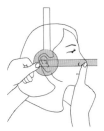

3. Align the arm of the goniometer that is to move with nares.

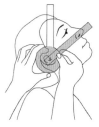

4. Ask your client to take their head as far back as possible, trying to get the back of their head to touch the top of their back. As the client does this, move the arm of the goniometer you have aligned with nares. Be sure to keep the stationary arm of the goniometer fixed. Take your measurement.

Measuring Lateral Flexion of the Neck with a Goniometer

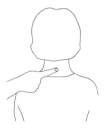

1. Locate the spinous process of C7.

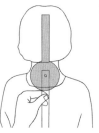

2. Locate the occipital protuberance and spinous processes of thoracic vertebrae.

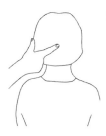

3. Position the center of your goniometer over C7, with the stationary arm over the spinous processes of thoracic vertebrae and the moveable arm over the occipital protuberance.

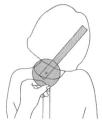

4. Instruct your client to keep their shoulders still and down as they move their head to try and get their ear to touch the shoulder on that side. Keep the moving arm in alignment with the occipital protuberance and take your measurement at the end of range. Repeat this on the opposite side.

Alternative Method of Measuring Lateral Flexion

Lateral flexion can also be measured using a goniometer as the therapist stands in front of the client.

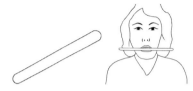

1. Start by asking your subject to hold a tongue depressor between their teeth. These are inexpensive and may be obtained from many pharmacies.

2. Position the goniometer parallel to the tongue depressor.

3. Ask your client to take their ear to their shoulder on the side at which you are holding the goniometer. Move the goniometer as they do this, keeping it parallel with the tongue depressor. Measure the number of degrees of lateral flexion when they reach the end of their active ROM.

Measuring Neck Rotation with a Goniometer

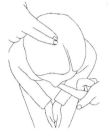

1. Locate the very top of the head and the acromion process.

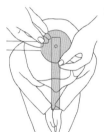

2. Position the center of your goniometer over the center of the head and the stationary arm over the acromion process. Position the moving arm of your goniometer over the tip of the nose.

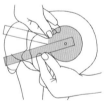

3. Ask your client to try and keep their chest and shoulder still as they turn their head to look over one shoulder. Move the stationary arm of the goniometer as they do this, keeping it aligned with the nose. At the end of range, take your measurement. Repeat on the other side.

Document your findings

Note the date.

Note the position of your client during the ROM tests.

Note what equipment you used.

Record your measurements.

For example
  • Flexion 50%
  • Extension 10%

  • Right rotation 20%
  • Left rotation 30%
  • Right lateral flexion 25%
  • Left lateral flexion 30%

Record anything else you think was significant.

For example, "client was unable to rotate to the right without shrugging the right shoulder."

Tip 4: Using a Tape Measure to Measure Cervical ROM

Flexion

Measure the distance from the chin to the sternal notch.

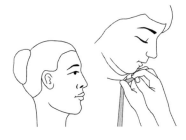

Lateral Flexion

Measure the distance from the mastoid process to the acromion process

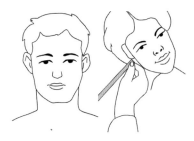

Extension

Measure the distance from the chin to the sternal notch.

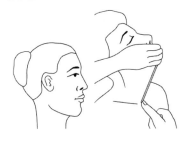

Rotation

Place a mark on your client's acromion process. Measure the distance from the tip of the chin to the acromion process (on the side to which the client rotates).

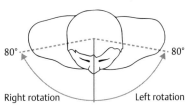

80°   80°

Right rotation   Left rotation

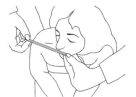

Tip 5: Documenting Your ROM Findings

Let us take the example of a client who comes to you with a stiff neck. You assess them, asking them to do the active ROM test, and then you decide on an appropriate treatment. Assuming that the goal of your treatment is to decrease their feelings of stiffness and/or increase their actual active movement, you will need to document the client's current limitation in ROM, as well as their posttreatment increase in ROM. Here are some ideas.

- One way to do this is to make a little sketch. It could be a small oval to represent a head, like the cartoons shown here.

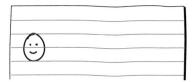

- Or, it could be a line, either superimposed over the sketch or simply on its own.

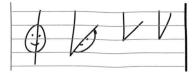

- Or, you could guesstimate in degrees the amount by which the range is decreased. For example, if rotation was decreased by what you thought was 5 degrees you could write –5 degrees with a line representing rotation.

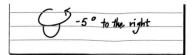

Experiment with different ways to document ROM findings until you find those that you are comfortable with and, importantly, which you will understand when you refer to your notes in the future.

Tip 6: Checking Quality of Movement

Sometimes a client is able to perform full ROM, yet the quality of their movement is poor. Maybe they wince or grimace as they perform the movement (another good reason to face your client when you carry out ROM tests) and yet are still able to perform it fully. Maybe they stop and start, taking their neck through its full range but with hesitancy. Or perhaps you simply get a sense of their caution, that they are guarding themselves. Hesitancy may be common following whiplash injuries, for example, when the tissues are healed, but the client is fearful of reinjury. A client with an inability to perform active cervical ROM fluidly could be described as having a "poverty" of movement. It is as important to document the quality with which a movement may be performed as it is to document the ROM attained, as this provides yet another piece of your assessment puzzle.

As with your documentation of the actual ROM, you will need to find a way to record the quality of movement in a way that you understand. "Poverty," "hesitancy," "guarding?," etc., could be useful. Notice that there is a question mark after "guarding." This is deliberate because we cannot know as a therapist whether someone is guarding themselves when they move their neck, as this is a subjective assessment of the movement we have observed.

Question: What might you record if you observe a client to have full range of active neck movement, yet in order to perform the movements the client keeps wincing?

In documenting *your* observations, would it be appropriate to write something like:

full movement—?pain

What do you think?

Tip 7: Documenting Discomfort

Many clients visit a therapist hoping to get relief from discomfort in their neck. If you are reading this as an experienced therapist, you will know that the words clients use to describe how they are feeling do not always involve the word "pain." Have you ever come across someone who says that their neck is "pulling," "tight," or that it "clicks"? Or someone who says they have a "sore" neck or that it is "a bit crunchy"? Can you remember whether you repeated the words used by the client, or whether, in response, you said something like, "So whereabouts is the pain?" It can be a challenge to avoid using the word "pain." It is a word bandied about, used to embrace a plethora of descriptive terms such as those listed above as well as "stiff," "aching," and "hurt." But why should it matter? Why not document your client's problem using the word "pain" as a generally descriptive term? Accurate documentation is important for several reasons. First, because if we use a patient's description of their symptoms as a baseline measurement against which we judge the effectiveness of our treatment, then it is important we do this accurately. "Pulling" or "crunching," for example, are descriptions of sensations which we are likely to want to lessen. If, following the treatment of a client with such symptoms, we ask them, "Has your pain diminished?" the answer will be meaningless. What we need to be asking is whether their "pulling" or "crunching" sensation has diminished.

Another important reason for using and documenting what clients say is that by doing so people feel that they are being "heard." This alone increases the chances of building rapport between the client and the clinician. A third reason for accurate recording of terms used is that this prevents the assessment water from getting muddied. If you start using the word "pain" too often to describe a client's symptoms, sooner or later the client will start using the word. This can lead to misdiagnosis and inappropriate treatment.

A final important reason for using the patient's exact terminology is that people tend to use similar words to describe similar diseases, and so having precise words can help with a more precise diagnosis. For example, and very generally, clients experiencing problems involving nerves might describe their symptoms as "sharp," "shooting," or "tingling," whereas those clients suffering bone or muscle problems might use words such as "deep," "boring," or "aching." Some of the words clients use to describe neck symptoms following whiplash can be very strange indeed, and it is important that as therapists we document whatever words our clients use in order to add to the collective understanding of how such conditions present in the clinical population. This concept is explored in depth in *Pain: The Science of Suffering* by Patrick Wall (1999).

TIP: A tip for helping you to avoid prompting your clients with use of the word "pain" is to write out some alternative questions. For example:

"Can you elaborate?"

"What sort of discomfort is it?"

"When did you first notice it?" (rather than "When did you first get the pain?")

"When you say it is uncomfortable, can you be more specific?"

Using these kinds of open-ended questions encourages the client to search for words that best describe their symptoms and can help you discover more about the nature of the problem.

Tip 8: A Differentiation Test

This next test is simple and rather crude but may help determine whether a neck problem is purely muscular, or whether there is an underlying skeletal/ligamentous component. It is a useful test because if you suspect that a client's problem may be due to the cervical vertebrae themselves, or due to the ligaments of these joints, it means that you are in a good position to refer your client to a physiotherapist, an osteopath, or a chiropractor for further investigation if the specific assessment of joints is outside your professional remit.

For this test, you will need to stand behind your client, which, as was noted in Tip 1 (p. 6), has certain disadvantages. However,

it is necessary for this particular test. This test relies on what your client says, so it is important to listen to the descriptive terms they use.

First, with your client seated, test their ROM by asking them to perform the movements of flexion, extension, lateral flexion, and rotation described in Tip 1 (p. 6). Observe the degree and quality of movement, and ask how the movements feel.

Document these findings. Remember from Tip 7 (p. 22) to identify the exact words the client uses to describe any discomfort, words such as "pulling," "pinching," "sticking," "catching," or "squashing."

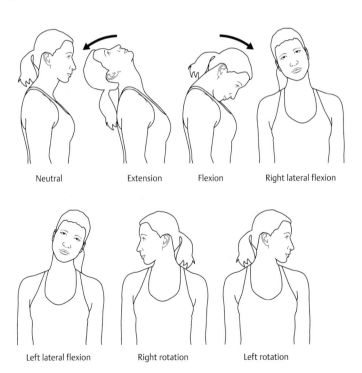

| Neutral | Extension | Flexion | Right lateral flexion |

Left lateral flexion   Right rotation   Left rotation

Second, still standing behind your seated subject, passively elevate their shoulders, supporting them under the elbow. Safeguard your own posture as you do this to avoid straining your back. Maintaining this position of passively elevated shoulders, ask your client to repeat the active cervical ROM, observe their movements, and again get feedback.

Passively elevating the shoulders takes some tension out of the muscles spanning the shoulder–neck region and reduces the pull on their connecting fascia. Therefore, if with passive elevation of the shoulders, pain/stiffness/discomfort is *reduced*, and ROM is *increased*, there is a strong likelihood that muscles such as upper trapezius, levator scapulae, or rhomboid minor are contributing to the client's problem. These muscles or their surrounding fascia, or both may be shortened.

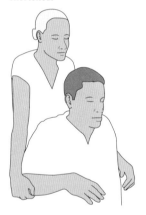

However, if there is little or *no difference* in pain/stiffness or discomfort, and *no increase* in cervical ROM, this suggests that the cervical vertebrae, their disks, or their ligaments are contributing to the problem. The rationale for this conclusion is that by reducing tension in the muscles spanning the shoulder–neck region, you would expect there to be a reduction in discomfort if it was originating from tension in these tissues. If there is no reduction in symptoms, the symptoms cannot be originating from these soft tissue structures (although it is likely that if there is an underlying joint problem, *some* muscular tension will develop, possibly a movement dysfunction also, and therefore the increased muscular tension and/or shortening of soft tissue will contribute in a minor way to the problem).

Another way to consider this is that if the problem exists in the joint, passively elevating the shoulders will make no difference: the joint still has to move. If anything, passively elevating the shoulders decreases muscular tension and allows the neck to move further. This may increase tension on the problem joint and can heighten the symptom. That is in fact what often happens: a client with a known cervical joint problem will report that the test mildly increases discomfort or makes no difference to the discomfort, whereas a client with muscular tension in the neck reports a decrease in symptoms—as one might expect when muscular "pull" is taken out of the equation, albeit slightly.

TIP: One way you could decide for yourself whether this is a useful assessment tool is to carry it out on people who you know have underlying bony or ligamentous problems yet are not contraindicated for assessment.

Passive elevation of the shoulders also lessens the tensional pull on scalenes during active rotation of the neck. Try this for yourself: Look over your right shoulder and as you do so, notice how the anterior left side of your neck feels. Next, ask a colleague to passively elevate your shoulders and repeat the movement. With passive shoulder elevation, do you notice less tension in your left scalenes on rotation of your head to the right?

Tip 9: Measuring Neck and Shoulder Distance

Another interesting assessment you can perform is to examine the distance between the widest part of a client's head and the widest part of their shoulders. The method by which this is done provides a helpful visual aid that can be used to help explain to clients the importance of maintaining correct neck alignment while they are sleeping.

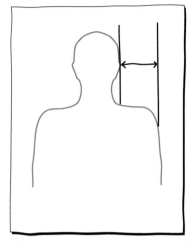

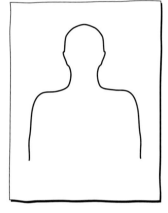

You will need a large enough floor space for your client to lie down and for you to kneel beside them. Take a large sheet of paper (or several smaller sheets fixed together) and ask your client to lie down on it in the supine position. Help get your client positioned so that their head and shoulders are on the paper. (You do not need their waist or lower part of their body on the paper, just their head and shoulders.) Next, draw around your client, keeping your pen perpendicular to the paper. Draw as close to the client's body as possible. Now ask your client to stand up.

Next, take the image you have drawn and measure the distance between the widest part of the client's head (i.e., at the level of the ears) and the widest part of their shoulders. Examine the distance between the head and the shoulders. Compare left and right sides. Measure the distance if you want. Are you surprised at how large this distance is? Is it the same on the left and right sides of the client's body?

This assessment gives both you and your client a visual understanding of the relationship between their head and neck. This information can be used to show your client how to keep their neck in alignment when sleeping on their side. For more information, please see Chapter 3, Tip 6 (p. 130).

Tip 10: Locating C7 on Yourself

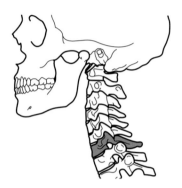

You no doubt remember having to learn anatomy as part of your therapy training, including the names given to groups of different vertebrae (cervical, thoracic, lumbar, sacral, coccygeal), and you may also have learned that these have letters and numbers assigned to them. Cervical vertebrae are assigned the letter "C" and numbered 1 to 7, from the top-down. The first cervical vertebra (also known as atlas) is referred to as C1 and the second (also known as axis) is referred to as C2. The seventh cervical vertebra—C7—is aptly named the *vertebra prominens* because it is the most prominent of the cervical vertebrae and it is a useful bone to be able to locate. Being able to locate this bony prominence gives us a point of reference when assessing and treating clients with neck problems. For example, we can use this point to document whether a tender spot is superior or inferior to C7 and thus be clearer as to the site of a symptom. Should you need to refer your client to another therapist, being able to describe symptoms in relation to this point may be helpful. For example: "Client reports posterior neck pain on rotation of the head to the right, specific to a point which is level with C7 but approximately 2 cm to the right of the C7 spinous process."

Sometimes a client reports a problem in their neck, yet on palpation, you discover the point the client is describing is in the high thoracic region. You know this because you have identified C7 and together you and your client have determined the place the client describes as being inferior to C7. So, being able to locate C7 is useful in order to get a more specific picture of where discomfort may be originating from or where symptoms may manifest.

Try locating C7 on yourself in order to gain confidence in palpating this bony prominence: Place your fingers on the back of your neck, flex your neck, and notice that the spinous processes of some vertebrae become prominent. As you move from C7 to C6 to C5, the spinous processes become less distinct and are therefore more difficult to differentiate from one another. In this position, are you able to determine that point on the back of your neck which feels most prominent? Whichever it is, this is likely to be the spinous process of your C7 vertebra.

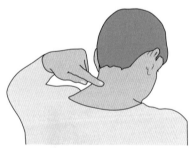

Tip 11: Locating C7 on a Client

C7 vertebra may be easily located with the client standing or seated. With your client in the prone position, it can sometimes be slightly trickier to identify.

Locating C7 on a Standing or Seated Client

Standing to the side of your client, observe their neck. In many subjects, there is a noticeable "bump" at the base of the neck, made more apparent when they look to the floor, flexing the cervical spine. This bump is C7. When you palpate the back of the neck, the spinous process of C7 is the most prominent. In clients who are very overweight or who have a dowager's hump—with an overgrowth of fatty tissue on the back of the neck—C7 can be harder to see. It seems obvious, but it will also be harder to see in people whose *vertebra prominens* have shorter, less prominent spinous processes.

Locating C7 on a Client in the Prone Position

When a client rests in the prone position, with their head and face in a neutral position rather than to one side, the neck extends slightly and the spinous processes of the cervical vertebrae approximate one another. With the neck in slight extension, it becomes less easy to distinguish individual vertebrae. Follow these simple steps to help you identify C7 in the prone position.

1. Standing at the head of the couch facing your client's head, place the thumb of your right hand where you think C7 might be.

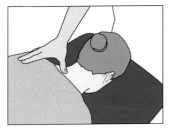

2. Place the thumb of your left hand where you think C6 might be.

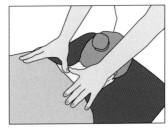

3. Keeping your thumbs in this position, ask your client to gently lift their head from the couch.

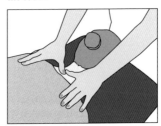

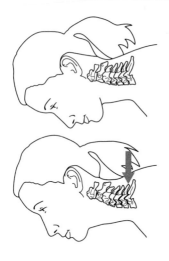

If your right thumb is on C7, you should feel the spinous process of C6 "disappear" beneath your left thumb. This is because the spinous processes of the cervical vertebrae approximate one another when the neck is moved into extension, making them more difficult to palpate. C7—at the cervicothoracic junction—remains relatively static. While you may feel this vertebra moves slightly, the movement will not be to the same degree as C6.

For a good reference in support of this method of identification, please see Shin et al (2011).

Tip 12: Getting Good at Locating C7

The shape and prominence of C7 varies considerably between subjects, and you may find that at first you are not sure whether you have correctly identified the vertebra. There are three ways to confirm you are on C7.

The best way to get good at palpating this bone—or any bony landmark—is simply to practice. Try to find it on a lot of different people. As the saying goes, practice makes perfect.

A second way to improve your skill is to place a mark on C7 with the client sitting, prior to palpation. Using a body crayon, place a dot over this vertebra, which will be more prominent when the client is upright, thus giving you a visual clue when it becomes less prominent as the client assumes the prone position. It is important to note, however, that the dot you mark on the skin with the client seated will not remain in the same position over the vertebrae when the client lies prone, as the skin and soft tissues will move and change as will the vertebrae themselves. Your mark will at least give you a *rough* indication of the lowest point of the cervical spine, and you can use this as a guide.

Thirdly, give this exercise your best attempt by following the steps in Tip 11 (pp. 27–28) and then, using the same client, deliberately place your thumbs in the *wrong* positions: place your right thumb over T1 (instead of C7) and your left thumb over C7 (instead of C6). Ask your subject to once again lift their head off the couch. Change back to the correct positions described in Tip 11—that is, with your right thumb on C7 and your left thumb on C6. Ask your client to lift their head. Compare the difference you feel beneath your thumbs in the "right" and "wrong" positions. By making comparisons between how different areas of the neck feel when you palpate C6 and C7, you can eventually decide which is the most *likely* location of C7. The most likely location when palpating in the prone position is when C6 "disappears" beneath your thumb.

Tip 13: Identifying Scalenes on Yourself

Scalenes are an interesting group of neck muscles because they may be responsible for referring pain to other parts of the body such as the medial border of the scapula (in the location of the rhomboids), the shoulder, and the upper limb. Nerves and blood vessels pass down to the upper limb by coursing through a small area which is bordered by the clavicle, ribs, pectoralis minor, and scalene muscles.

therapists find that by decreasing tension in these muscles—through stretching, massage, trigger point work, or repositioning of the head and neck through exercise, for example—symptoms of thoracic outlet syndrome are alleviated in some subjects. Attaching to the first and second ribs, scalenes are also important muscles of respiration. Being able to identify and to palpate them is therefore useful in assessing for muscular tension.

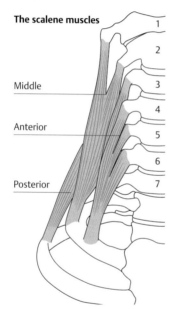

The scalene muscles

1
2
Middle
3
4
Anterior
5
6
Posterior
7

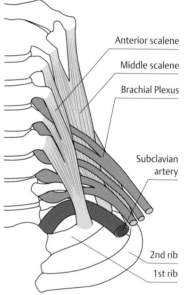

Anterior scalene

Middle scalene

Brachial Plexus

Subclavian artery

2nd rib

1st rib

Compression of the blood vessels or nerves in this area of the neck leads to a range of upper limb symptoms collectively known as *thoracic outlet syndrome*. There is controversy surrounding whether tension in scalenes may contribute to thoracic outlet syndrome. Some

Some people feel anxious about having their neck palpated, especially the anterior aspect. To gain confidence with assessing this sensitive area, follow these steps and practice identifying your own scalenes.

STEP 1 Facing a mirror, first identify the two muscles which are *not* scalenes. Draw your mouth downward and locate the flat sheet of the platysma muscle that resembles a turtle's neck. Note that the tendons of this muscle are at the lateral ends of your clavicles.

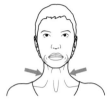

STEP 2 Relax your mouth and locate sternocleidomastoid. This muscle rotates the head and neck to the opposite side: the right sternocleidomastoid rotates the head and neck to the left; the left sternocleidomastoid rotates the head and neck to the right. Practice rotating your head one way and then the other until you are sure you have identified this muscle.

TIP: When you gently pinch the muscle at its base where it originates on the sternum and clavicle, you will feel it contract. For example, rotate your head to the left and note that you can feel your right muscle contract.

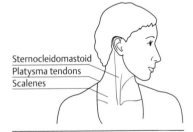

Sternocleidomastoid
Platysma tendons
Scalenes

STEP 3 Locate the *position* of scalenes. These are located between the tendons of platysma and the sternocleidomastoid muscle. That is, your right scalene muscles are located between the right platysma tendon and your right sternocleidomastoid muscle; your left scalene muscles are located between the left platysma tendon and your left sternocleidomastoid muscle.

STEP 4 Now that you know the *region* in which to look and palpate for scalenes, let us identify them for sure. Face the mirror and place your right fist against your forehead. Gently push your head into your fist and notice that your scalenes (on both sides) become prominent as they contract. You will see them above your clavicles and just lateral to the sternocleidomastoid on each side, but not as lateral as the tendon of platysma, the "turtle" neck muscle.

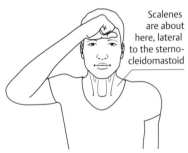

Scalenes are about here, lateral to the sternocleidomastoid

The answer is to palpate them while they contract. This is where it is useful to revise some muscle functions. Both scalenes and the sternocleidomastoid bring about neck flexion and so both contract when you press your forehead into your fist as described. However, the right scalenes do *not* contract when you turn your head to the left (whereas the right sternocleidomastoid does) and the left scalenes do *not* contract when you turn your head to the left (whereas the left sternocleidomastoid does). We can use this information to differentiate between scalenes and the sternocleidomastoid.

Differentiating between Scalenes and Sternocleidomastoid

STEP 1 Locate both the right sternocleidomastoid and the right scalenes by observing for and palpating these as they contract on resisted neck flexion. You will see the muscles "appear" when you press your head into your fist, and you can palpate and "feel" the increase in tone, demonstrating that both muscles have contracted. Next, you need to do something that is a bit tricky.

STEP 2 Place your right hand against the right side of your head and resist right rotation while palpating *both* sternocleidomastoid and scalenes. It may work best if you place your left thumb on the sternocleidomastoid and your left forefinger on the scalenes.

You will feel that one of these muscles contracts on right rotation, but the other does not. That is, as you turn your head to the right, you can feel an increase in tone in only one of the muscles. The right scalenes contract on rotation of the head to the right, but the right sternocleidomastoid does not. Unlike the sternocleidomastoid, scalenes rotate the head and neck *to the same side*, whereas the sternocleidomastoid muscles rotate the head and neck *to the opposite side*. If you have correctly identified your right scalene muscles, you will feel them contract on both neck flexion and rotation of the head to the right.

Tip 14: How to Observe Scalenes on a Client

Scalenes are deep muscles and should not be apparent when you observe a subject at rest, from the front, although you may see them in clients with certain respiratory disorders (remember these are muscles of respiration) where these muscles have become hypertonic due to the extra workload imposed on them. You may see these muscles in subjects with very low body fat. As you might expect, in such people many muscles become more discernible, not just scalenes. However, in a normal, healthy adult, scalenes should not appear prominent. Look closely to see whether one side appears more pronounced than the other. This may indicate an increase in tone on that side. Such an increase in tone may correspond with symptoms on that side of the body.

Secondly, you could locate these muscles on a client in the same way that you located them on yourself. Ask your client to face you and to place their own fist against their forehead and gently resist forward flexion. Observe your subject as you instruct them to perform gentle, resisted neck flexion. Like when you tried this exercise yourself, you should see scalenes on either side of the client's neck, between the tendon of platysma and the sternocleidomastoid muscle.

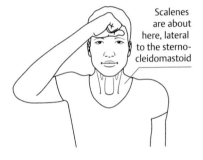

Scalenes are about here, lateral to the sternocleidomastoid

Question: What if you wanted to identify scalenes with your client in the supine position?

Simply ask them to gently lift their head from the couch and scalenes will be activated and will become prominent. Lifting the head from the couch requires flexion of the neck and because the head is being lifted against gravity, it is not necessary for the client to press their forehead into their fist.

Tip 15: How to Palpate Scalenes on a Client

There are two ways to do this.

1. **Palpating scalenes with your client seated:** Stand behind your client and gently palpate the anterior of their neck using light, fingertip touch.

TIP: Use only one hand. Rest your other hand gently on the client's shoulder. The reason for this is that it can be unnerving to have someone stand behind you with both hands on your neck, albeit for the purposes of assessment and within a professional capacity. Having both hands around the neck, even with light fingertip touch, could make some clients anxious.

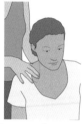

Locate your subject's clavicle and keep your fingers on or superior to this bone.

Ask your client to place one of their fists gently on their forehead and to gently press their forehead into their fist. As you know, both scalenes and the sternocleidomastoid will contract when they do this. Palpate along the clavicle, superior to this bone, feeling for the contraction in scalenes.

From practicing on yourself as described in Tip 13 (pp. 30–32), you now know that only scalenes contract ipsilaterally on rotation. That is, the right scalene contracts on rotation of the head to the right (whereas the sternocleidomastoid does not) and the left scalenes contract on rotation of the head to the left (whereas the left sternocleidomastoid does not). By asking your client to turn their head to the right, for example, you should now be able to identify their right scalene muscles: you should know that they can be palpated superior to the clavicle, close to the bone, in between the sternocleidomastoid muscle and the tendon of platysma.

2. **Palpating scalenes with your client supine:** It is sometimes easier to palpate scalenes with a subject supine than it is with them seated. Standing at the head of the couch, using one hand only, once again palpate your subject's neck superior to the clavicle, between the sternocleidomastoid and the platysma tendon. Ask your client to lift their head off the couch. Once again, the scalenes will contract and you should be able to identify them as an increase in tone beneath your fingertips.

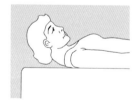

For more information about these fascinating muscles and tips on how to treat trigger points in them, turn to Chapter 2, Tip 18: Treating Scalenes (pp. 104–105).

Tip 16: **The Tongue Test**

In his book *Do-It-Yourself Shiatsu*, Wataru Ohashi (1977) says that if you ask a client to stick out their tongue, you can determine which side of their neck is "tight" by the direction the tongue is pointing. A tongue pointing to the right indicates tension in the right side of the neck; a tongue pointing to the left indicates tension in the left side of the neck. Ohashi explains that this is due to muscles pulling on the tongue. What do you think? Are you tempted to try this form of assessment? Although Ohashi does not state which muscles are responsible for observed

tongue deviation, we know that omohyoid is a strange little strap-like muscle connecting the superior angle of the scapula with the hyoid bone and, as you may remember, the hyoid bone is the bone at the front of the throat anchoring the tongue. As you will learn from Tip 17, the shoulder is related to the neck, so it would be interesting to observe whether there is any tongue deviation in clients with shoulder problems. Are you brave enough to include this as a form of assessment?

Tip 17: Appreciating the Neck/Upper Limb Relationship

Place the fingers of your right hand on the back of your neck, in the center, along the spinous processes of your cervical vertebrae. Now abduct your left arm. Notice that you can feel subtle movement beneath your fingers. Swap hands, this time palpating your neck with the fingers of your left hand while also abducting your right arm. You are likely feeling an increase in tone in trapezius (where it inserts to a soft tissue structure called the *ligamentum nuchae* running down the spinous processes of the cervical spine), which you may remember spans the posterior of the neck and attaches to the spine of the scapula and which contracts to help bring about movement of the scapula.

So why is this important? The neck and shoulder are connected via a huge array of soft tissues. While the neck is the focus of this section, it is well known that we cannot treat parts of the body in isolation. (Many would argue that we cannot treat *the body* in isolation—the mind must be addressed also.) When a client comes for treatment of a neck problem, assessment of the shoulder is useful—many would argue essential. Existing or previous shoulder problems may contribute to a current neck problem and both of these parts of the body will need to be addressed if there is to be a successful resolution.

Therefore, while there are time constraints on how long you can assess and treat a client, it is worth considering a shoulder assessment if the neck problem you are treating remains unresolved. In such cases, it is useful to enquire and to reflect on how your client is using their upper limbs, because it is impossible to compartmentalize the body in real life, as you know. Levator scapulae is a muscle which, when you learn more about it in the next tip, helps make this point clearer.

Tip 18: What Are "Knots" in the Neck Region?

If you are used to providing massage for your clients, you are likely to have felt some areas of the neck and shoulder to be bumpy or knotty. Experienced therapists know that when "trigger points" are pressed, they elicit a kind of "grateful pain." It may be that you have come across a trigger spot, a small, localized area of tension that when pressed produces this kind of pain. It is important to remember that not all areas of palpable tension are trigger points.

First, they could be normal bony anatomy. Look at a model skeleton and observe how the ribs protrude posteriorly. Though not as likely in the cervical region, it is possible that an area of tension you can feel is in fact a rib. Although rare, a small percentage of the population have a cervical rib that is palpable anteriorly.

Secondly, the area of tension could be normal muscular anatomy. Consider levator scapulae. This muscle originates on the transverse processes of the upper cervical vertebrae and inserts on the superior angle of the scapulae. Notice how it twists back on itself. Could the "knots" you sometimes feel in this region actually be normal muscular anatomy rather than tense tissues?

If you suspect levator scapulae *does* contain trigger spots, and that it is not just normal muscular anatomy you can feel, reading Chapter 2 will be helpful as it provides tips on how you can position your client in various ways to gain better access to this muscle.

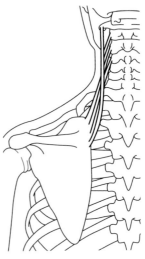

Thirdly, there are other explanations for palpable lumps, such as lipomas, tumors, or scar tissue, for example. The purpose of this section is not to teach diagnostics, and if you have any doubt as to whether the lump you have found is a trigger point or normal musculoskeletal anatomy, you should refer your client to their doctor.

Tip 19: The Importance of Suboccipitals

Attaching to either of the first two cervical vertebrae, the four small muscles at the base of the skull that are collectively known as suboccipitals are responsible for rocking and tilting the head. Feel the flicker of your own suboccipitals by placing your fingertips gently beneath the occiput. Now roll your eyes in a circle. Can you feel your suboccipitals flickering? One of these muscles is known as rectus capitis posterior minor and is particularly curious because it has a high proportion of muscle spindles. Muscles with a high proportion of spindles are involved in proprioception. So atrophy of this muscle in clients following injury (such as whiplash) may be significant and may contribute to a reduced sense of balance.

Rectus capitis posterior minor is also important because it is connected to the dura mater of the brain via a layer of fascia. Tension and the development of trigger points in suboccipitals may be one explanation for tension headaches, as increased tension is transmitted to the dura via this fascial connection.

Further, as injury or atrophy of suboccipitals could affect balance, these muscles may contribute to hamstring tension. For a discussion of this point, and further information, see McPartland et al (1997) and Moseley (2004).

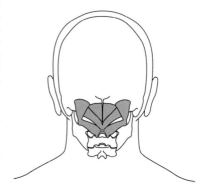

Tip 20: Palpating Suboccipitals

It is difficult to effectively palpate these muscles as they lie deep to trapezius and the thick fascia of the posterior of the neck. One way to palpate the posterior neck is with the client prone. However, if they try to turn their head, they need to lift it, extending the neck; muscles of the posterior neck become tense, thereby making palpation difficult. An alternative is to position your client supine. Practice palpating the posterior neck in these positions and see which works best for you.

- Client prone, you at the head of the couch.

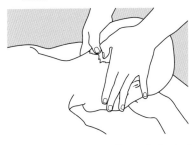

- Client supine, you standing at the head of the couch with your hands either side of the client's neck.

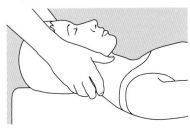

- Client supine, you facing your client with your hands either side of their neck.

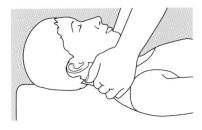

- Client supine, you standing at the head of the couch, cupping the base of the skull.

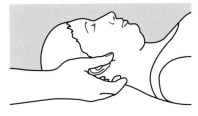

- Client lying on the side, you standing behind them.

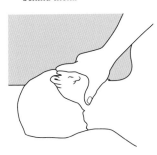

Tip 21: Client Perceptions of Pain

In Tip 7: Documenting Discomfort (p. 22), you read about the importance of documenting the terminology used by clients to report their symptoms. It is also important to consider how a neck problem impacts on the activities of daily life for a person—how it affects their work, family life, and participation in hobbies. Based on the *Oswestry Low Back Pain Disability Questionnaire* (Fairbank et al 1980), the Neck Disability Index (NDI) is a questionnaire designed to measure self-perceived disability resulting from neck pain. A similar questionnaire was designed by the team at Northwick Park Hospital in England and is called the Northwick Park Neck Pain Questionnaire (NPQ) (Leak et al 1994). Both of these questionnaires comprise a series of questions which cover pain intensity, personal care (washing, dressing, etc.), lifting, reading, headaches, concentration, work, driving, sleeping, and recreation.

The purpose of such questionnaires is to help identify the level of disability that the neck problem represents to a client. The results serve as a baseline marker and enable practitioners to identify whether their interventions are reducing the overall level of disability that the client perceives themselves to have.

Examining the validity of these questionnaires for use with patients suffering from Whiplash Associated Disorders (WAD), researchers Hoving et al (2003) noted that the questionnaires omitted emotional and social items judged to be important to patients. Nevertheless, you could use the subheadings from the questionnaires as a prompt when assessing your own clients to determine how their neck condition impacts on their daily life. A sample prompt sheet has been provided for you below.

Activity	Comments
Personal care	
Lifting	
Reading	
Headaches	
Concentration	
Work	
Driving	
Sleeping	
Recreation	

Tip 22: Neck Disability Index

Vernon and Mior (1991) developed a questionnaire called the Neck Disability Index (NDI). They considered how a neck problem affects people in terms of what most people do on a daily basis, during an average day. To assess this, they devised a series of questions, which they grouped into 10 sections:

- Section 1: Pain Intensity
- Section 2: Personal Care (Washing, Dressing, etc.)
- Section 3: Lifting
- Section 4: Reading
- Section 5: Headaches
- Section 6: Concentration
- Section 7: Work
- Section 8: Driving
- Section 9: Sleeping
- Section 10: Recreation

By asking people to answer the questions within each section of the questionnaire, clinicians get a better idea of how a person's neck problem affects their ability to cope with the activities of daily life. The answers to these questions are assigned numerical values, which mean they can be tallied and used to come up with an overall score. This makes it possible to use the NDI to help measure change over time, to determine whether a particular intervention has been useful.

Question: I'm not a doctor or neck specialist, so is it still worth using the questionnaire?

One way of utilizing this questionnaire would be to help clients identify where they *do not* have a problem, which aspects of their daily life are *not* affected by their neck pain. Helping clients to identify pain-free times of their day and the activities they can perform pain free can be very empowering. Another way you could use it is to prompt your own thinking and to trigger lines of enquiry. For example, if "Section 4: Reading" is scored highly, you could explore whether it makes a difference in which position your client reads—sitting on a high-backed chair or sitting up in bed, for example—or you could ask whether it makes a difference how heavy the book is or whether they hold it on their lap or on a book rest. A client who reports pain in their neck from reading journal articles while sitting at a desk may not get the same pain when they hold the lightweight journal in front of them. The kind of information that can be generated by using this questionnaire is invaluable in helping clients to find ways to manage their pain.

If you want to try this questionnaire, you could practice by using it with a family member or friend who you know has had neck problems. Ask them to read the simple instructions and then complete the questionnaire. You will need to read the instructions at the end of the questionnaire that tell you how to create a "score" (see pp. 44–45).

Once you have read the instructions and understood how to use the NDI, you could use the following table to record the scores for five people you know have a neck problem. Compare the numerical results. Those with a higher percentage score are classed as having a higher level of neck-related disability. Do you agree with this? Would you say that your subjects who rated more highly have a higher level of disability? Another useful comparison might be to examine five people you know have had a common neck-related disorder such as whiplash or a trapped nerve.

Practicing with the Neck Disability Index Score		
Subject	Neck Disability Index Score	Comments
Subject 1		
Subject 2		
Subject 3		
Subject 4		
Subject 5		

Neck Disability Index

Information for clients: This questionnaire has been designed to help me understand how your neck pain has affected your ability to manage in everyday life. Please answer every section and in each section mark ONE box that applies to you. If you consider that two or more statements in any one section relate to you, please mark the box that most closely describes your problem.

Section 1: Pain Intensity

☐ I have no pain at the moment.

☐ The pain is very mild at the moment.

☐ The pain is moderate at the moment.

☐ The pain is fairly severe at the moment.

☐ The pain is very severe at the moment.

☐ The pain is the worst imaginable at the moment.

Section 2: Personal Care (Washing, Dressing, etc.)

☐ I can look after myself normally without causing extra pain.

☐ I can look after myself normally, but it causes extra pain.

☐ It is painful to look after myself and I am slow and careful.

☐ I need some help but can manage most of my personal care.

☐ I need help every day in most aspects of self-care.

☐ I do not get dressed, wash with difficulty, and stay in bed.

Section 3: Lifting

☐ I can lift heavy weights without extra pain.

☐ I can lift heavy weights but it gives extra pain.

☐ Pain prevents me lifting heavy weights off the floor, but I can manage if they are conveniently placed, for example, on a table.

☐ Pain prevents me from lifting heavy weights, but I can manage light to medium weights if they are conveniently positioned.

☐ I can only lift very light weights.

☐ I cannot lift or carry anything.

Section 4: Reading

- ☐ I can read as much as I want to with no pain in my neck.
- ☐ I can read as much as I want to with slight pain in my neck.
- ☐ I can read as much as I want to with moderate pain in my neck.
- ☐ I cannot read as much as I want to because of moderate pain in my neck.
- ☐ I can hardly read at all because of severe pain in my neck.
- ☐ I cannot read at all.

Section 5: Headaches

- ☐ I have no headaches at all.
- ☐ I have slight headaches, which come infrequently.
- ☐ I have moderate headaches, which come infrequently.
- ☐ I have moderate headaches, which come frequently.
- ☐ I have severe headaches, which come frequently.
- ☐ I have headaches almost all the time.

Section 6: Concentration

- ☐ I can concentrate fully when I want to with no difficulty.
- ☐ I can concentrate fully when I want to with slight difficulty.
- ☐ I have a fair degree of difficulty in concentrating when I want to.
- ☐ I have a lot of difficulty in concentrating when I want to.
- ☐ I have a great deal of difficulty in concentrating when I want to.
- ☐ I cannot concentrate at all.

Section 7: Work

- ☐ I can do as much work as I want to.
- ☐ I can only do my usual work, but no more.
- ☐ I can do most of my usual work, but no more.
- ☐ I cannot do my usual work.
- ☐ I can hardly do any work at all.
- ☐ I cannot do any work at all.

Section 8: Driving

- ☐ I can drive my car without any neck pain.
- ☐ I can drive my car as long as I want to with slight pain in my neck.
- ☐ I can drive my car as long as I want to with moderate pain in my neck.
- ☐ I cannot drive my car as long as I want to because of moderate pain in my neck.
- ☐ I can hardly drive at all because of severe pain in my neck.
- ☐ I cannot drive my car at all.

Section 9: Sleeping

- ☐ I have no trouble sleeping.
- ☐ My sleep is slightly disturbed (less than 1 h sleepless).
- ☐ My sleep is mildly disturbed (1–2 h sleepless).
- ☐ My sleep is moderately disturbed (2–3 h sleepless).
- ☐ My sleep is greatly disturbed (3–5 h sleepless).
- ☐ My sleep is completely disturbed (5–7 h sleepless).

Section 10: Recreation

- ☐ I am able to engage in all my recreation activities with no neck pain at all.
- ☐ I am able to engage in all my recreation activities, with some pain in my neck.
- ☐ I am able to engage in most, but not all of my usual recreation activities because of pain in my neck.
- ☐ I am able to engage in a few of my usual recreation activities because of pain in my neck.
- ☐ I can hardly do any recreation activities because of pain in my neck.
- ☐ I cannot do any recreation activities at all.

How to score the Neck Disability Index

Each of the 10 sections is scored separately (0–5 points each) and then added up (max. total = 50). Note that while there are six questions within each section, the first question scores 0. If the first statement is ticked, the section score is 0; if the last statement is ticked, it is 5.

EXAMPLE:

Section 3: Lifting

- ☐ I can lift heavy weights without extra pain (0.)
- ☐ I can lift heavy weights, but it gives extra pain (1).
- ☐ Pain prevents me lifting heavy weights off the floor, but I can manage if they are conveniently placed, for example, on a table (2).
- ☐ Pain prevents me from lifting heavy weights, but I can manage light to medium weights if they are conveniently positioned (3).
- ☐ I can only lift very light weights (4).
- ☐ I cannot lift or carry anything (5).

If all 10 sections are completed, double the client's score to get a percentage figure.

Example 1: if you add up the client's scores and this equals 30, then 30 × 2 = 60. So their percentage disability is 60%.

Example 2: if their total score is 12, then 12 × 2 = 24. So their percentage disability is 24%.

The higher the percentage, the more the neck problem is affecting the client in their daily life.

If I have a client who cannot complete all of the sections, can I still use the questionnaire? Yes. If you were treating a client who cannot drive, for example, they will not be able to complete Section 8.

To calculate the score when a section cannot be completed or has been omitted, divide the patient's total score by the number of sections completed times 5:

$$\frac{\text{PATIENT'S SCORE}}{\text{\# OF SECTIONS COMPLETED} \times 5} \times 100 = \% \text{ DISABILITY}$$

Example 1

If 9 of 10 sections are completed, and the score is 30:

$$\frac{30}{9 \times 5} \times 100 = 66.66\% \text{ disability}$$

$$\frac{30}{45} \times 100 = 66.66\%$$

Example 2

If 9 out of 10 sections are completed and the score is 22:

$$\frac{22}{9 \times 5} \times 100 = 4.8\% \text{ disability}$$

Tip 23: Postural Assessment Reminder

Here is a reminder about some of the things you may choose to look for in a postural assessment of the head and neck.

Ear level	Head and neck tilt
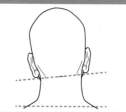	
Uneven ear level could mean that the client's head and neck are laterally flexed to one side, or simply that they have one ear positioned higher than the other. Where the latter is the case, clients often know this because they report finding it difficult to get glasses to sit properly.	Clients observed to have lateral neck flexion when resting are likely to have shortened muscles on the side to which they are flexed, notably levator scapulae, scalenes, sternocleidomastoid, and the upper fibers of trapezius on that side of the body.

For full descriptions of what to look for in a postural assessment of the neck region, see Johnson (2012).

Head and neck rotation	Cervical spine alignment
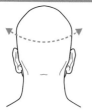	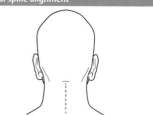
Can you see more of one side of your client's face than the other? More of their jaw or eyelashes on one side? A client who appears to be rotated to the right when relaxed could have shortened scalenes and levator scapulae on that side, and an increase in tone in the sternocleidomastoid on the left side of their neck.	It is also worth checking to see whether the cervical spine itself appears to be in alignment. Does it appear vertical? Are there any marks or swelling present? How do the paraspinal muscles running up the back of the neck appear—are they very prominent? Are muscles on both sides even in tone?

Notice from these illustrations how small lateral deviations in the neck significantly alter the angle between the upper cervical vertebrae and the skull. Where there is a decrease in angle (a), tissues will be shortened; where there is an increase in angle (b), they will be lengthened. These findings may help explain a client's symptoms and will help inform your treatment.

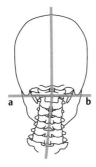

The forward head posture describes a type of posture in which the head is carried in advance of the body. The head weighs about 5 kg (11 lbs) and should rest directly over the thorax so that the weight of the head is supported by the slightly lordotic curve of the cervical vertebrae. However, as your head moves forward, muscles on the posterior of your neck (levator scapulae, for example) have to work extremely hard. This is fine for everyday movements of the head and neck, into and out of flexion and extension, but is not good when the head remains in the forward position. When the head rests in the forward position, posterior cervical muscles are required to maintain this position and begin to fatigue, and tissues become lengthened and stressed. This is one of the reasons people with this type of posture experience pain in the neck and shoulders.

As muscles of the posterior of the neck lengthen and fatigue, they weaken. Anterior neck muscles may become shortened and weak, as they are also held in a less than optimal position. The result is altered head and neck biomechanics, and this has a knock-on effect to other parts of the body. Other parts of the spine are then strained as they struggle to counterbalance a heavy head that is being held too far forward and is not being supported through the midline of the body. It is for this reason that many therapists argue that treatments to the thorax and lumbar spine have short-lived effects if the neck and head positions also are not addressed in people with thoracic and lumbar problems. We do not know whether the maintenance of a forward head posture *causes* low back pain, but it seems reasonable to assume that such a posture could certainly *aggravate* dysfunction in the lumbar region.

Head position	Cervicothoracic junction
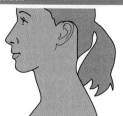	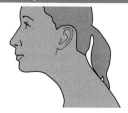
Does the head appear to sit over the thorax or is it pushed forward? Such a posture causes levator scapulae to become hypertonic as it struggles to maintain and move the head in a less than optimal manner, often having to work isometrically. In such a posture, the suboccipitals are also stressed as they work to tilt the head backwards so that the eyes are facing forward, and often clients with such a posture experience tenderness when the suboccipitals are palpated and massaged.	Look at the position of C7. Does there appear to be an abnormal overgrowth of fatty tissue here? This is frequently observed in people with forward head postures where there is a raised portion of tissue over the C7/T1 junction.
	Question: What causes this deposit of fatty tissue? It is not clear whether this is hormonal (it is frequently seen in women) or the result of an altered posture and less efficient neck–thorax biomechanics.

Head position	Clavicles
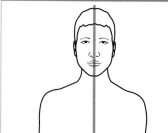	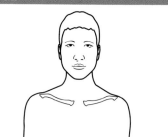
Does the head sit comfortably over the thorax? Is the nose aligned over the manubrium? Is any rotation or lateral tilt that was observed posteriorly also evident in an anterior observation?	Are the clavicles even in both height and orientation? How sharp is the angle they form from the sternoclavicular joint? The smaller the angle, the higher the shoulder on that side. Do they have smooth contours?

Muscle tone	Shoulder level
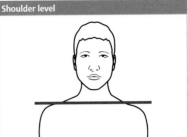	
Can you see the scalene muscles or the sternocleidomastoid? Is there an increase in tone in muscles on one side of the neck compared to the other? Prominence in the appearance of these muscles can indicate a forward head posture or chronic respiratory condition.	It is impossible to separate the neck from the shoulder region, so any observation of the neck should also take into account the position of the shoulders both anteriorly and posteriorly and when the client is viewed from the side.

Tip 24: **Functional Strength Testing**

Cervical strength is usually tested by the examiner holding the client's head still while the client attempts to move their head through each of the cervical ranges, one at a time. The examiner notes the strength the client exerts, whether this appears to fall within a normal range for someone of their age, whether there are any obvious weaknesses or differences between left and right sides, and whether such resistance provokes any of the client's symptoms. However, such tests tend to fall within the remit of physiotherapists, osteopaths, chiropractors, and sports therapists rather than massage therapists.

One of the simplest and safest methods to assess the strength of neck muscles is to ask a client to perform active neck movements against gravity. The table here shows four different test positions and the muscles that are required to bring about the movement in each position. A client should be able to repeat the movement six to eight times. Being able to repeat the movement only one or two times indicates weakness in one or more of the muscles associated with this movement.

Position	Movement	Muscles responsible
Supine	Neck flexion	Sternocleidomastoid
		Scalenes
		Longus colli
		Longus capitis
Prone	Neck extension	Splenius capitis
		Suboccipitals
		Longissimus
		Levator scapulae
		Semispinalis (capitis and cervicis)
		Upper fibers of trapezius
Side lying	Lateral flexion	Trapezius
		Levator scapulae
		Scalenes
		Sternocleidomastoid
		Splenius capitis
Supine	Rotation	Sternocleidomastoid
		Splenius capitis
		Semispinalis cervicis
		Suboccipitals
		Trapezius

Chapter II

Neck Treatment

Chapter 2 **Neck Treatment**

If you have been struggling to achieve the results you want when treating clients with neck problems, or if you simply want some additional treatment ideas, consider using some of the techniques described in this chapter, the theme of which is *less is more*. Many of the tips you will find here encourage you to relax, to be focused, and to explore the subtle changes that occur in the body as a result of very light touch. When you try a technique different from the one you have been using, you tend to work cautiously and are therefore likely to sense gentle, minor movements of the body and in the body tissues. Although subtle, these changes can be positive and are often profound. You may discover that by doing less, you facilitate an "allowing" of relaxation, and this helps stimulate the repair process. You might achieve greater success with a client by adopting a lighter touch than if you try to "worry" away tension, pain, stiffness, or discomfort with an overuse of manual techniques.

Other tips in this section encourage you to consider changing the position in which you treat a client, and some tips provide ideas for treating specific muscles such as suboccipitals, scalenes, and sternocleidomastoid.

If you are reading this as a massage therapist, you may be pleased to know that there is evidence to show that massage is effective for the treatment of neck pain. For examples of research papers examining the use of massage for neck pain, see Sherman et al (2009) and Ezzo et al (2007).

Tip 1: Less Is More

Have you ever treated a client with a neck problem that at first seemed to improve, but for whom, over time, your results began to plateau? Have you ever found yourself repeating the same kind of treatment with a client, hoping that things would improve while being secretly frustrated that you were not making better progress? Perhaps there have been times when you have utilized every technique you know, exhausting your entire armory of skills, yet the improvements you were hoping for were not forthcoming. It can be tricky to know quite what to do in such situations.

Usually there is *some* progress, and so it is tempting to keep going, to keep providing the same treatment or advice, hoping that there will be a breakthrough sometime soon and that your client will turn up for a session saying, "Hey! After that last treatment I wasn't expecting anything different and yet when I woke up on Sunday I could look over my left shoulder again!" After all, we frequently tell our clients that it can take weeks or even months to resolve a problem, that a neck problem which has built up over many years is not likely to be resolved in a just a few treatment sessions. So with our client's best interests at heart we begin with what we imagine will be a program of treatment, some point in which we will identify a time when the client will no longer need us, a time when they will be able to manage their condition themselves, or their symptoms will resolve entirely. Yet you may have experienced a situation where you at first seemed to make good progress, with the client reporting immediate relief from symptoms, but with successive treatment sessions there was less and less improvement. If this happens toward the end of a successful treatment program, that is good, and one might expect the degree of change to be less with time anyway. There is often

a gradual tailing off of treatment as the client's condition improves, and they are naturally weaned off us. But if this slowing down in improvement occurs before a reasonable relief from pain, stiffness, or other troubling symptoms, it can be frustrating for you as a therapist. There is always the feeling that we ought to do more, that we *want* to do more. The good news is that, if the treatment you currently provide for a client is proving ineffective, there are many things you could do instead of continuing with the same treatment.

1. *Reassess your client*: You could reassess your client, right from the beginning, reevaluating their range and quality of movement, and asking questions to determine whether anything has changed in their work, hobbies, or lifestyle that may be relevant to the symptoms they are currently experiencing. The client may be doing something that they do not consider affects their neck, and so has not thought of telling you about it. This could be something quite simple, like deciding to watch an entire series of their favorite TV drama or to read *War and Peace* cover to cover or to knit a king-size blanket. All of these examples require the maintenance of a static neck posture, which, for most of us, is not a good thing. Static postures are likely to aggravate some neck problems. Being able to identify an ongoing aggravating factor is very helpful, so reassessment is useful. The tips in Chapter 1 provide over 20 further ideas for how you might assess your client. Could any of these be useful to you?

2. *Consult a colleague*: With permission from your client, you could enlist a colleague to carry out the reassessment. Perhaps a colleague will identify something you have missed? They may use a different handhold or phrase a question in such

a way as to elicit a different reply; they may perform a test with a subtle change or palpate more firmly (or less firmly). It is always worth asking for a "second opinion" because a colleague sometimes has a different "take" on things. Observing how another therapist performs a neck assessment can be a valuable learning experience in itself.

3. *Brainstorm*: Maintaining the confidentiality of your client, you could brainstorm the problem with other therapists, asking for their advice. Someone might suggest an assessment, treatment, or technique you had not considered and which could prove helpful. Perhaps a colleague has even treated a client with a similar condition? In what ways was it similar? In what ways did it differ? What did they do that was helpful?

4. *Explore internet forums for information*: The value of sharing information about treatments that have proved effective cannot be overestimated. Sometimes this information can be gleaned from colleagues or you may find it on an internet forum. While you do need to be discerning in which pieces of information to accept, forums are a useful way of sharing information and much can be learned from reading the comments posted by forum users.

5. *Consider referral*: You could refer your client to a more experienced practitioner or to a different health professional entirely. It may be that your client has a condition that is not treatable with your particular therapy, or a condition of which you are not aware. Having to refer a client shows you are putting their needs before your own and should be regarded as a strength rather than a weakness.

Question: How long should you wait before referring a client to another practitioner?

This is a difficult question to answer definitively as this depends on the nature and severity of the symptoms as well as on any protocols set out by your governing body or insurance provider. Your answer must depend on what you consider likely to give your client the best treatment outcome.

6. *Avoid hands-on treatment entirely*: If you feel that you have correctly assessed your client, there is no need for referral, and you do not wish to discuss treatment options with another therapist, another option is for you to do less with the neck, instead of more. At the extreme end of the scale, you could avoid any hands-on treatment entirely. Consider all of the aftercare tips provided in Chapter 3 and select those that you feel might be appropriate for your client. Use the information in these tips to provide your client with the means to self-manage their condition while you remain on hand to offer advice.

7. *Reduce your pressure*: Sometimes, we risk over-treating. That is, we try to do too much, too soon, perhaps because we are so eager to help. Or we use too much pressure during a particular treatment session. Sometimes the client enjoys the sensation of deep pressure; sometimes it provides the results we seek; sometimes we feel that by "working" an area it will improve, especially if at the assessment stage, we discover there to be a palpable increase in muscle tone. If you are providing massage, try lightening your touch by half, so that the pressure of your strokes is halved. Then lighten the depth of your touch by half again. If you are a therapist used to using a lot of pressure, it can be difficult to change your approach, especially if you have achieved good results in the past with deep tissue massage. Yet sometimes, if we step back, take a breather, and choose to work with

less effort, our treatment outcomes improve. This may be because by working more slowly, more gently, with far more patience, we become attuned to the nature of the problem. By sitting very still, with a lightness of touch that is only just perceptible, the clients with whom we are working may begin to find the emotional space to help bring about the healing they need.

8. *Change your focus*: You could consider treating a different part of your client's body altogether. Sometimes, working away from the problem area rather than directly over it brings about unexpected and positive results. An example of how this might work is provided in Tip 2, where you will learn how to facilitate an increase in neck range of movement by treating the shoulder and not the neck.

Tip 2: **Gentle Shoulder Traction to Increase Neck Mobility**

Let us put this "less-is-more" approach into practice immediately. A good example of how a less-is-more approach might work is to imagine you are going to treat a client with tension in muscles of their neck. You know that the neck and shoulder cannot really be isolated anatomically, owing to the large number of structures which connect these two parts of the body to each other and also connect them to the face, skull, upper limb, and thorax.

Question: What are some examples of structures which connect the neck and shoulder?

Omohyoid is a strap-like muscle connecting the scapulae to the hyoid bone at the front of the throat; the upper fibers of trapezius connect the scapulae, clavicle, cervical vertebrae, and occiput; the brachial plexus is a group of nerves in the armpit originating from the cervical region; the fascia of the deltoid links the fascia of the chest and neck and arm; skin of the shoulder is continuous with the skin of the neck, chest, and face.

Hence by reducing tension in the shoulder you may help to reduce tension in the neck via these interconnected structures. Stretching often alleviates muscular tension but instead of stretching the neck, how about gently stretching some of the tissues connecting the shoulder and the neck, without touching the neck itself at all?

This does not have to be the *only* treatment you provide—you could also stretch the neck, massage the neck, and use any of the other techniques familiar to you. It is good, however, sometimes to start with something very simple, and experience just how beneficial this can be *before* moving on to more direct techniques.

Question: If the results are positive after this simple stretch, is there a need to do further treatment to the neck?

You may decide that there is no need to do further work, to apply further techniques. Sometimes it is best to let the treatment take effect and to reassess a client the following day or in a few days' time. It can be surprising how effective these nondirect techniques can be.

Question: Are there any clients for whom this is specifically contraindicated?

Yes, this would not be appropriate for clients with shoulder subluxation or dislocation, with known hypermobility syndromes, or recent trauma to the neck or shoulder.

To perform a simple shoulder–neck stretch, read the question concerning contraindications and if you feel that it is appropriate for your client, follow these steps.

STEP 1 Position your client comfortably in the supine position and stand to one side of the treatment couch. Avoid use of a pillow beneath the head if possible. Gently take hold of the client's arm, keeping it close to their body. In a moment, you are going to apply *gentle* traction to the shoulder joint, avoiding traction to the elbow and forearm. It is for this reason that you need to find a way to clasp the arm above the elbow joint. You may find that it helps if your client positions their hand on the inside of your own arm, as if holding your tricep, or for you to hold the arm with the elbow flexed. Whichever handhold you settle on, it is important that you avoid tractioning the elbow: you want your "pull" to be focused more proximally at the shoulder joint. Practice with different handholds until both you and the client feel comfortable.

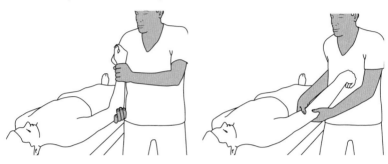

Question: Why should I avoid tractioning the elbow?

When you traction the upper limb, force is transmitted through the soft tissues (skin, fascia, muscle, tendons, ligaments, nerves, blood vessels, etc.). *If you hold the upper limb at the arm* (i.e., the bicep/tricep region) and apply gentle traction, the force of this gentle stretch is transmitted through the shoulder, and through the soft tissues connecting the shoulder to the neck. *If you hold the limb below the elbow* (at the forearm region), this force is transmitted through the soft tissues of the elbow, through the arm, and then through the shoulder and neck, with decreasing stretch being felt in the shoulder and neck. *If you hold the upper limb by the hand*, the force of the stretch is transmitted through the wrist, forearm, elbow, arm, shoulder, and finally some of the soft tissues of the neck. There are two reasons for placing your hands superior to the elbow. The first is that you want the focus of the stretch to be in the soft tissues of the shoulder and the neck. Holding the limb superior to the elbow achieves this. The second is to avoid tractioning the elbow joint itself, or indeed any of the tissues distal to this, because even though the force you apply is *extremely* gentle with this stretch, in many people it can feel uncomfortable, especially where there is tension in tissues of the upper limb. There *are* techniques which involve handholds distal to the elbow, but for the technique being described here, try your best to hold the limb so that your stretch is focused on the shoulder and neck regions only.

TIP: With a colleague, practice holding each other's arm at the wrist, at the forearm, and then as shown below, and compare how it feels when you are the recipient of the stretch as it is performed with each of the different handholds.

STEP 2 Keeping the client's arm close to their body, apply *gentle* traction and sustain this. Maintain your position. Tell yourself to relax. Discourage your client from talking but, of course, encourage them to let you know if they feel uncomfortable and stop the traction if they report discomfort. As you maintain the traction, see if you can get a sense of the client relaxing. Can you also get a sense of the tissues of the arm and shoulder "releasing"? Relaxation and release may take a little time as the client settles into the position, acclimatizes to the technique, and allows themselves to "let go."

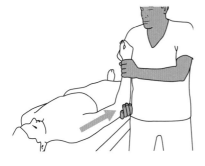

STEP 3 For some clients, this very simple shoulder stretch may be enough to provide some relief for a stiff neck, as the soft tissues joining both structures gradually release. However, some subjects may get more benefit if they *slowly* turn their head away from you—simply rolling it to the opposite direction only as far as they feel comfortable—once you are in position and have applied the stretch. It is important that you apply traction *first*, before the client turns their head away from you. In this way, it is the client who is in control of how far they rotate, and therefore in control of how much tension is placed on the soft tissues of their neck and shoulder. Can you see how, if the client were to rotate *before* you applied traction, it would be you, the therapist, who was in control of the stretch? If you were to perform the stretch that way, with the client turning their head first, before you applied traction, you could potentially stress the tissues too much.

STEP 4 After a couple of minutes, gently release both positions: encourage the client to return their head to neutral (if they had rotated it away from you), and relax the traction. Gently return the client's arm to rest on the treatment couch and repeat the technique on the opposite arm.

Question: Is this technique the same as a myofascial release (MFR) arm pull?

No, when performing a MFR arm pull you hold the hand and wrist, with slight supination of the forearm. MFR arm pulls can be very beneficial and it is worth training in MFR if this is something that interests you.

Tip 3: Two Techniques Using a Towel to Increase Range of Movement

Here is the first of two very gentle techniques that employ the use of a towel to increase range of movement in the neck. For each technique, you will find it helpful to use a towel that is not too thick, about the size of a hand towel.

Technique 1

Position your client in the supine position with the towel beneath their head. When they are comfortable, grasp each end of the towel as shown and use it to gently move the client's head from side to side, letting the head roll one way and then the other. Be sure to move the head *slowly*.

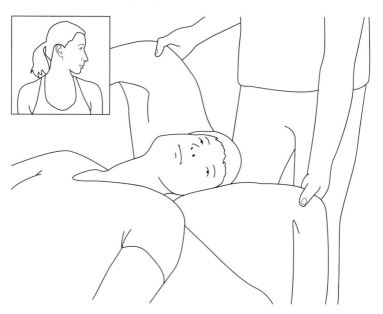

TIP: Avoid the temptation to lift the head from the couch because when the head is lifted, some clients have an instinctive tendency to tense their neck muscles. Many clients feel safer, and are therefore more able to relax, when they can feel their head supported by the couch.

The advantage of this technique is that it facilitates rotation without you having to touch the client's head and face with your hands. Some clients enjoy receiving the sensation of passive neck rotation but dislike having oily hands on their face or hair. It is worth experiencing this technique for yourself to help determine what speed of motion left to right and right to left feels most appropriate.

Question: Are there any clients for whom this movement is contraindicated?

For most of the clients who could receive neck massage, this technique is safe. However, as it involves a rotatory movement, be cautious when using this technique with clients suffering from inner ear disorders such as Ménière's disease.

Technique 2

You can modify the previous tip so that instead of facilitating rotation, you facilitate lateral flexion of the neck. To do this, simply alter the position into which you take the head, taking care to get feedback from the client because, as you lengthen and perhaps stretch one side of the neck, you passively compress the opposite side of the neck.

TIP: Keep only the neck in lateral flexion for a short time because muscles on the shortened side sometimes cramp.

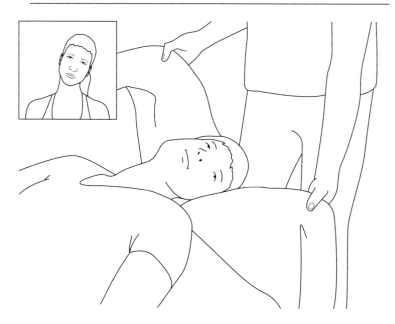

Tip 4: Releasing the Posterior Neck Tissues with Gentle Passive Stretch

In their excellent book, *The Myofascial Release Manual*, Manheim and Lavette (1989) describe how to release tension in the soft tissues of the back of the neck in a manner with which you may not yet be familiar: MFR. If you are reading this as a massage therapist, it is important to realize that the technique described in this tip should be performed without the application of a massage medium. The technique is very gentle, yet even so, use of oil or wax would make it difficult for your fingertips to get enough purchase on the skin to facilitate the relaxation in tissues. Therefore, when practicing this technique, do so without any oil or wax, but on dry skin only.

STEP 1 With your client in the supine position, make sure you too are comfortable at the head of the couch. Once you have performed this technique once, you will have a better idea of whether or not you need to change your treatment position, from standing to sitting, for example. Manheim and Lavette (1989) suggest that you position your client in such a way that you have adequate support for your elbows on the treatment couch.

STEP 2 Begin by gently cradling the client's head, gaining their confidence and encouraging them to relax. Start stroking the back of the neck slowly and when you are ready, choose one of the four handholds shown in the illustration on the following page.

STEP 3 Apply very *gentle*, sustained traction, just enough for you to feel some resistance in the tissues. Hold this position and wait. Wait until you sense the tissues release. Once you feel this release, either stop or apply gentle traction again.

TIP: Practice using each of the four handholds, perhaps on different subjects, and decide with which hand position you feel most comfortable. You could practice all four handholds on the same person, but remember, you do not want to fatigue your client by overtreating them. You are likely to discover that, as with other techniques, given the variety of human anatomy, different handholds suit different clients.

Alternative handholds

- Cupping the head at the base of the skull with one hand and applying slight overpressure with the other.

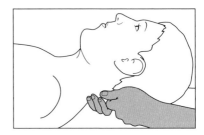

- Cupping the base of the skull with both hands.

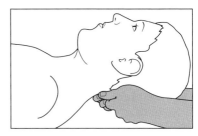

- Cupping the base of the skull with one hand and placing the other on the client's shoulder.

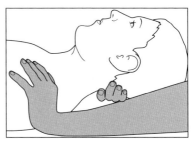

- One hand on the client's sternum, against their skin, and the other hand cupping the base of the skull. (You may feel that this is inappropriate for some clients.)

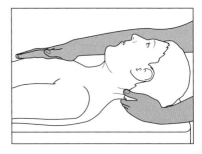

Tip 5: Be Careful with Overpressure in Neck Flexion

A better understanding of anatomy can help you to become a better therapist. A good example of how knowing your anatomy can help inform your treatment is when you consider the form and function of the top two cervical vertebrae. C1 and C2—atlas and axis as they are called—have facet joints orientated at a different angle to the facet joints of other cervical vertebrae. In vertebrae C3–C7, the facet joints are slanted at an angle. The facet joints between atlas and axis are also slanted, but to a lesser degree.

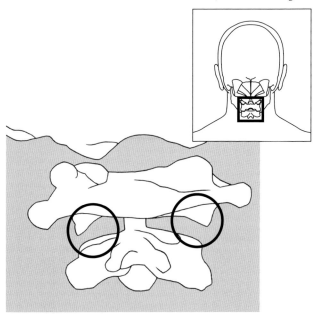

Relatively speaking, the atlantoaxial facet joints are orientated more horizontally than the facet joints in the rest of the cervical spine. So how does that information help inform our practice?

Well, flexion of the head and neck with overpressure is often performed to stretch the soft tissues on the back of the neck. Yet in flexion, the facet joints of the atlas and axis bones are compressed. Flexion with overpressure, as is common in neck flexion stretches, may put excessive strain on the facet joints between these top two cervical vertebrae. This is not a problem in most healthy individuals, but may pose a risk when treating clients with osteoporosis or those who have a pathology affecting their facet joints. In such cases, there is a good argument for avoiding both active and passive stretches involving overpressure in flexion of the head and neck. Alternative stretches may be safer. The next tip describes a method for stretching the posterior neck tissues *without* flexion.

Tip 6: Using a Towel to Facilitate a Passive Neck Stretch

For those clients who enjoy the sensation of a slightly stronger stretch than those described in Tip 4 (pp. 64–65), this next technique may prove useful. It is easy to perform but note that the strength of the stretch as perceived by the client is partially influenced by how you hold the towel and the height of your treatment couch.

STEP 1 Position your client in the supine position with a small hand towel beneath their head. Make sure they have removed any earrings. Check the position of the towel. It should be placed so that when you lift it, it hooks nicely into the occipital bone, the base of the skull. Grasp the towel as close to your client's face as possible. This is important because if you grasp the towel too far away from the face, the stretch

feels quite different to receive and instead of gentle traction you end up tilting the head back a little into extension.

STEP 2 Slowly and carefully start to bring your arms toward you, gently stretching the muscles of the posterior neck.

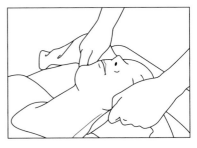

TIP: One trick is to use the very edge of the towel, rather than a towel edge that has been folded over, as this gives a better "hook" into the occiput.

TIP: Your clients cannot hear you when receiving this stretch as the towel covers their ears. It is therefore useful to agree beforehand on a simple signal to indicate if the stretch feels too strong and the client wishes you to stop. One such signal is simply for them to raise their hand.

Tip 7: Changing the Treatment Position

One of the things you might consider in order to provide variety for both yourself and your clients, and as an experiment when working with clients with whom you are not progressing as quickly as you would like, is to change the position in which the client has been receiving treatment. Consider changing from prone to supine, or from supine to seated, or from seated to side lying, for example. Tips 8, 9, 10, and 11 provide ideas on how you might utilize different treatment positions to your advantage. To begin with, here is a summary of the advantages and disadvantages of each position.

Prone	
Advantages	**Disadvantages**
• Allows easy access to the back of the neck. • Tissues of the back of the neck can be seen and assessed visually, facilitating treatment to muscles such as levator scapulae, trapezius, and paraspinals. • Makes linking the back of the neck to the shoulders and thorax easy using massage strokes. • The therapist can stand at the head or at the side of the treatment couch. • Can be a useful position when treating clients who are severely kyphotic. • Can be useful when needing to treat the base of the occiput, insertion of sternocleidomastoid or the back of the head.	• Tissues of the anterior neck cannot safely be treated; tissues on the side of the neck may be more difficult to treat in this position. • Not always suitable for clients who feel claustrophobic. • Communication is more difficult: Clients cannot always hear the therapist in this position; therapists cannot always hear the client. • Can make treating clients with a very lordotic neck or kinked neck difficult, unless the client is able to chin tuck comfortably. • Can be uncomfortable for clients with low back problems unless a pillow is placed beneath the stomach. • Is not appropriate for clients in later stages of pregnancy, or clients whose anterior is affected by discomfort, recent injury, or surgery (e.g., abdominal bloating, anterior knee pain, mastectomy). • Some clients dislike the temporary mark left on the face or forehead from the face cradle. • Resting in the prone position too long, some clients discover their nose starts to run.
Supine	
Advantages	**Disadvantages**
• Tissues of the anterior and side of the neck are easy to access, facilitating treatment to scalenes and sternocleidomastoid. • Although the posterior neck tissues cannot be seen, they can be palpated in this position and are sometimes easier to palpate this way owing to the decrease in tone resulting from a relaxed head position. • Can be very useful when treating clients who cannot comfortably lie prone. • Makes linking the front and sides of the neck to the chest easy using massage strokes. • Can be a useful position when there needs to be an ongoing dialogue between the client and the therapist.	• May be more difficult to access tissues of the posterior neck. • Posterior neck tissues cannot be seen. • May be uncomfortable for clients with an exaggerated kyphotic curve. • Can be uncomfortable for clients with lumber problems unless they rest with hips and knees flexed or a bolster beneath their knees. • Is contraindicated in later stages of pregnancy.

Side Lying	
Advantages	**Disadvantages**
• It makes the side of the neck that is uppermost easy to access. • Can be very useful when treating clients who cannot easily or safely lie prone or supine, such as in later stages of pregnancy. • Tissues can easily be passively shortened or passively lengthened in this position, facilitating access to deeper structures. • Makes linking the side of the neck to the shoulder easy using massage strokes.	• The client has to swap sides during treatment and this can interrupt the flow of the session. • Can be difficult for the client to find a comfortable position for the arm on which they are resting. • May not be suitable for clients with shoulder problems who could find resting on their shoulder painful.
Seated	
Advantages	**Disadvantages**
• It is a very useful treatment position for when you want the client to be more engaged with the treatment they are receiving or when it is important for there to be an ongoing dialogue. • Can be very useful when treating clients who cannot easily or safely lie prone or supine, such as in later stages of pregnancy. • Facilitates access to the front, sides, and the back of the neck.	• The client may be less relaxed than in a lying position. • Tissues of the neck are under more tension when the client is seated than in other treatment positions. • Unless a face cradle is available, there is an increase in tone in muscles of the neck in the seated position as these work to support the head, even when the client attempts to relax.

Tip 8: Five Ways to Access the Neck in the Prone Position

1. *Chin tuck:* One of the ways you can gain better access to the back of the neck is to ask your client to tuck in their chin when they are resting in the prone position. By doing this they actively reposition their head into a more flexed position, thus lengthening the tissues on the posterior of the neck and helping to slightly gap the vertebrae posteriorly. This is especially helpful when treating clients with an excessively lordotic neck, a kinked neck, or with a dowager's hump—a fatty overgrowth of tissue that makes accessing the tissues of the posterior neck tricky at times. Clients may choose to do the chin tuck while resting with their face in a face hole or face cradle, or they may chose simply to rest their forehead on their hands. Whichever method they choose, this repositioning helps you gain access to the posterior neck, but remember that in this chin tuck position the posterior neck tissues are lengthened and under slightly more tension than when a client rests prone.

2. *Using a sponge to passively retract scapulae:* When a client rests prone, without the aid of any support, their shoulders fall naturally into protraction. Placing a large sponge, a small rolled up towel, or a tiny cushion beneath the client's shoulder as they rest in the prone position has the effect of passively retracting the scapula and in doing so passively shortens some of the tissues linking the neck and the shoulder. Passively shortening these tissues can help you to gain access to deeper tissues. To prove this for yourself, try both positions. Have your client lie facedown in the prone position, their shoulders allowed to fall forward, into protraction. Massage the upper fibers of trapezius. How does this muscle feel to you? Is it malleable, yet quite firm? Next, reposition your client by gently inserting a bath sponge, for example, beneath one of their shoulders. Now massage the upper trapezius. Can you feel how much softer the tissues feel now they have been passively shortened? See if you can palpate more deeply, identifying levator scapulae, the strap-like muscle running from the transverse processes of the top three to four cervical vertebrae and inserting onto the superior angle of the scapula. Can you identify this muscle which is often lengthened and feels "twangy"?

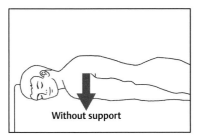

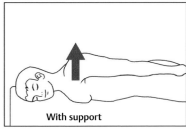

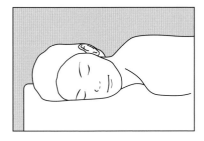

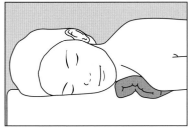

TIP: Avoid drawing the client's shoulder into too much horizontal extension as this can cause an uncomfortable stretch on the anterior of the shoulder. Some clients experience temporary pins and needles in their fingers due to temporary compression of nerves or vascular structures in the arm.

3. *Using your thigh for support*: If you do not have access to a support such as a towel or large sponge, you can position yourself as shown and passively abduct the arm, retracting the scapula. Sit on the edge of the treatment couch and gently support the client's arm in abduction, allowing it to rest on your thigh. You may feel that this is not an appropriate treatment position for all clients.

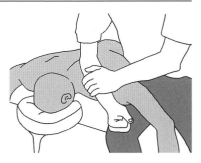

4. *Working with the shoulder elevated*: Another position you could try if you have not already is to position the client with their shoulder in elevation. While this passively shortens the soft tissues crossing the neck and shoulder joints, the disadvantage is that this position can trigger cramping or feelings of impingement in the supraspinatus muscle of some clients. This is because muscles sometimes cramp when passively shortened. It would therefore not be appropriate when treating someone with supraspinatus tendonitis or a torticollis.

TIP: This position also facilitates palpation of the scalenes on the anterior neck.

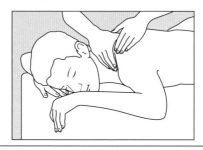

5. *Opening up the posterior region by increasing flexion*: Many therapists choose to use a treatment couch with an adjustable face cradle. Providing that the client is comfortable, you can experiment with facilitating varying degrees of neck flexion, thus facilitating better access to the back of the neck. This is helpful when working with clients who are very kyphotic, those who are very overweight and may have rather large necks, or those with a dowager's hump.

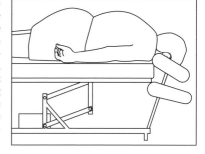

The following table compares the advantages and disadvantages of each of the five ways to access the neck in the prone position. Once you have had a chance to experiment, add your own notes. Do you agree or disagree with any of these points? What could you add?

Advantages	Disadvantages
Active or Passive Chin Tuck	
• Enables access to posterior neck tissues. • Good for treating clients with short necks or with a lot of fat in the neck region.	• Some clients feel squashed or claustrophobic. • If performed actively, difficult to maintain position for long periods without fatigue.
Passive Scapula Retraction with Sponge	
• Facilitates access to deeper structures such as levator scapulae.	• Some clients feel uncomfortable with one shoulder retracted. • Uncomfortable for clients with tight anterior shoulder muscles.
Passive Scapula Retraction Using Thigh	
• Facilitates access to deeper structures such as levator scapulae. • Therapist does not need any extra equipment to bring about the retraction.	• May be considered too intimate a position for some therapists/clients. • An uncomfortable treatment position for some therapists. • Some clients feel uncomfortable having one shoulder passively retracted in this way. • Uncomfortable for clients with tight anterior shoulder muscles.
Position 4: Passive Scapula Elevation	
• Facilitates access to deeper structures such as levator scapulae.	• Can trigger temporary spasm in upper fibers of trapezius and levator scapulae in some cases. • Not appropriate for treatment of shoulder impingement syndromes.
Position 5: Passive Neck Flexion	
• Enables access to posterior neck tissues. • Good for treating clients with short necks or with a lot of fat in the neck region.	• Not all clients feel comfortable with their head in this slight downward position. • Addition of a face cradle makes it harder to access lower regions of the back from the head of the couch (e.g., with effleurage) when incorporating neck treatments into a back massage.

Tip 9: Five Treatment Techniques with Your Client in the Prone Position

1. *Pulling into the occiput*: This is useful to help lengthen posterior neck tissues as you drag your fingers toward you, bringing about gentle traction on the skin, which sometimes draws the head into slight flexion. Or, alternatively, simply cradle your fingers beneath the occiput and wait to sense the subtle changes in pliability of the tissues against your fingertips.

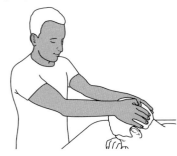

2. *Gentle gripping of posterior neck muscles*: In the prone position, it is easy to gently grip the tissues of the back of the neck and ever so gently pull them upwards, away from the spine. This can feel very relaxing providing you avoid pinching the skin too tightly.

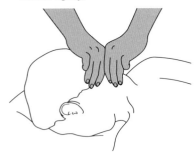

3. *Gentle static pressures to trigger spots*: If you are able to identify a trigger spot, it can be relieved with gentle, static pressure. If using your thumbs as shown below, be careful where you position your fingers. It can be tempting to rest them on the sides of the client's neck and jaw as shown below, but this can feel unpleasant for some clients. Note that if you are on a trigger spot, discomfort should resolve within about 60 seconds. If the spot continues to be painful, release your pressure. Be cautious when treating trigger points of clients with known neck pathologies, and avoid pressure to the vertebrae in osteoporotic subjects.

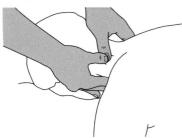

Experiment with different massage mediums. Notice that if you use oil, it can be difficult to get a purchase on the muscles in order to pull them gently toward you. One tip is to practice without any massage medium at all. How does your client feel if you simply pull and hold the tissues? Does it matter where you stand in relation to your subject?

Perhaps you have located a trigger point in the trapezius. Such points are easily treated in the prone position. You could treat the point as shown here or you could treat it with the shoulder in passive retraction as shown in Tip 8 (pp. 70–73). As you apply gentle pressure to the trigger spot, discomfort should start to dissipate. Avoid pressing too hard. Remember the theme of this chapter is "less is more."

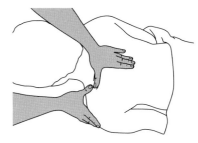

4. *Short, caudal strokes*: Small, longitudinal strokes can be applied from the client's head to the base of their neck (i.e., in caudal direction).

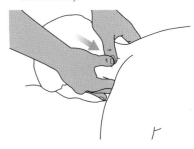

When treating in this way, be careful with the positioning of your fingers. Avoid

gripping the sides of the neck at the same time you are stroking downward, toward the shoulders; avoid using your fingers for leverage when applying thumb pressure. It may be necessary to flex your fingers, especially if you have large hands or when treating a client with a small neck. Compare stroking the neck with reinforced thumbs to stroking with alternate thumbs. Which feels best for you?

5. *Gentle transverse stretch using digital pressure*: Alternatively, reinforce one of your fingers as shown here, either to apply gentle, static pressure to a trigger point or to gently roll the skin and tissues transversely. Remember, you do not necessarily need to "rub" the tissues back and forth. This can irritate a point of discomfort rather than alleviate it. Instead, practice gently pushing the tissues away from you, allow for there to be a little traction on the skin, and wait to see if you can feel the tissues "creep" and release.

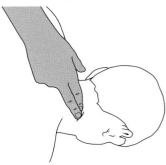

The following table summarizes uses for these five prone-position techniques.

Uses of each technique

1. Pulling into the occiput:
   - Acclimatizing the client to your touch.
   - Starting and ending a treatment.

2. Gentle gripping:
   - Passively stretching neck extensor muscles and fascia without moving joints of the neck.
   - Palpating for trigger spots.

3. Static pressures:
   - Alleviation of trigger points in neck extensor muscles with neck muscles relaxed.

4. Short, caudal strokes:
   - Soothing tissues after deactivation of trigger points.
   - Applying localized longitudinal stretch to neck extensor tissues.

5. Transverse stretch:
   - Passively stretching neck extensor muscles without moving cervical joints.
   - Localizing stretch of tissues to a specific spot.

Tip 10: Tips for Treating the Neck in the Supine Position

Treating clients in the supine position gives you the opportunity to treat all regions of the neck, and later tips provide specific ideas for how to treat scalenes, sternocleidomastoid, and occipitals in this position. Neck retractions, an exercise you will find described in Chapter 3, Tip 7 (pp. 131–133) can sometimes work better with the client in this position.

Some techniques work best when you remove the pillow, yet some clients may feel more comfortable with a neck support in the form of a small rolled up towel, especially if they have an increased cervical lordosis. Conversely, you may wish to facilitate a decrease in such a lordosis by placing a small towel beneath the head.

When a client is supine, their neck is in a neutral position. Some clients may feel more comfortable if they are allowed to rest in slight neck flexion, although this can make treatment more difficult for you, and you may find that you need to lower your treatment couch considerably.

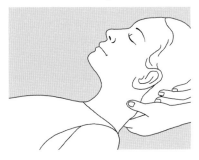

The supine position enables you to gently lift and cradle the head, to turn it gently side to side, something many clients find very soothing.

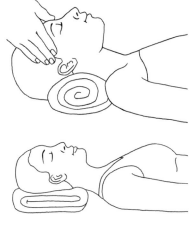

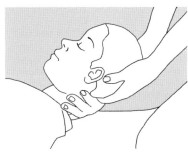

TIP: Experiment by role-playing with a colleague. When playing the therapist, give the instruction to "relax and let go" while holding the head as shown here. Then say, "again, relax and let go." See if you can identify the point at which client relaxes on both the first and the second instructions.

Techniques you can use with your client in the supine position include passive depression of the shoulders unilaterally or bilaterally (a), gentle stroking of the neck (b), and passive neck stretches with the head and neck being taken gently into lateral flexion (c).

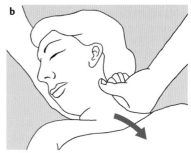

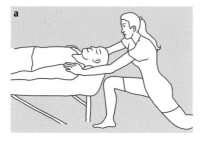

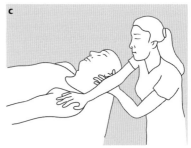

Additional Techniques in Supine

In addition to these last three techniques, at the beginning of this chapter you learned how gentle shoulder traction could enhance a neck stretch, and you were introduced to three neck stretches using a towel with your client in the supine position (one rotatory, one lateral, and one cephalad). You also learned that useful myofascial stretches can be applied with a client in supine. Later you will learn how to release suboccipital muscles using your fingertips and how to treat sternocleidomastoid and scalenes, some of the techniques applied in supine. Once you are familiar with these techniques, you could return to the following table and tick those techniques you have tried and circle those you want to practice again.

Technique	1	2	3
1. Gentle shoulder traction 			
2. Passive neck rotation with a towel 			
3. Passive lateral flexion with a towel 			
4. Passive (cephalad) stretch using a towel 			

Technique	1	2	3
5. Myofascial release of tissues			
6. Fingertips to suboccipitals			
7. Bilateral depression of shoulders			
8. Unilateral depression of shoulders			

Technique	1	2	3
9. Passive lateral stretch			
10. Longitudinal stroking			
11. Gentle stretch to anterior tissues			
12. Treating sternocleidomastoid			
13. Treating scalenes			

Remember, these are only some of the techniques you could use. If you are a qualified therapist, you may already be using some or many of these. If you are a student, there may be some you have not tried before. All of these can be interspersed with any techniques you are already using and with facial massage and massage to the anterior of the shoulders and the chest.

An Experiment in Focus

Let us focus now on just two techniques, depression of the shoulders and compression of trigger points in the upper fibers of trapezius. As an exercise, practice with a colleague and spend 5 minutes on each side of the neck using only these two techniques. See if you can answer the following questions.

1. Depression of the shoulders:
   - As you depress the shoulders one at a time, which feels easier to move, the left or the right shoulder? Does your subject sense any variation?
   - Does it matter where you place your hands, on the top of the shoulder at the head of the humerus or more anteriorly?
   - Does it matter which part of your hand you use to apply the depression?
   - How does it feel when you keep your palm in the same place but change the orientation of your fingers? Is this better or worse for your wrists as a therapist?
   - How does it feel to slowly depress one shoulder and to hold it in gentle depression for 20 seconds?
   - Finally, what happens if, as you gently depress the shoulder, your subject turns their head away from you? Do they experience a stretch or is this uncomfortable?

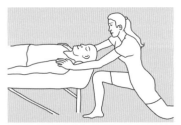

2. Applying gentle pressure to the trapezius on one side and palpating for trigger points:

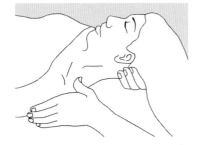

   - What happens if you gently compress a point and then use your other hand to slowly move your subject's head away from the point, tensioning the tissue. Is this relieving for your client or is it making them uncomfortable?
   - How does your thumb feel, comfortable or strained?
   - Can you discover any trigger points? Where are they? Are these lateral, close to the shoulder, or closer to the neck? Or do they fall in the middle of these upper fibers of trapezius, between the distal end of the clavicle and the neck itself?
   - How easy is it for you to compress the upper fibers of trapezius in this position? Do you feel that in order to access the trigger points properly you need your client to be in a position other than supine? Or can you access some of the points in this position?

Note that there are no right or wrong answers to these questions, and you and your colleague may have different experiences.

Use the following table to record your experiences.

Shoulders feel equal to depress?	Yes/No
Best position to place hands	
Best part of hand to use	
Finger orientation?	
Sustained depression feels...	
Sustained shoulder depression with active head movement	
Location of trigger points	
Compression of triggers with active head movement	
Thumb pain	Yes/No

Tip 11: **Tips for Treating the Neck in the Side-Lying Position**

Experimenting with a Pillow

This position can be useful in helping to "open up" the neck region, providing access to the lateral side of the neck. It requires some experimentation to discover the best use of a pillow with your client in the side-lying position. Using a pillow can help make your client comfortable but can hinder access to the whole of the back of the neck. Sometimes it is difficult for a client to rest in this position without their arm and shoulder getting squashed. Also, not all clients can lie on both their left and right sides equally well. They may be more comfortable on one side than on the other, so you cannot always expect to be able to treat both sides of the neck in this position. It is a useful position for treating pregnant clients or those for whom resting prone or supine is uncomfortable.

TIP: Remember that if your client is in the side-lying position, you may need to offer them a pillow or bolster for support between their legs or beneath the knee that is uppermost.

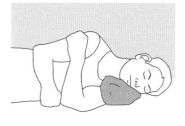 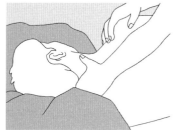

Passive Abduction of the Arm in the Side-Lying Position

Some therapists like to passively abduct the arm of their client as shown here. This has the effect of passively shortening some of the soft tissues spanning the shoulder and the neck and can therefore facilitate access to deeper structures. Not all clients are able to relax and "give" you their arm in this manner.

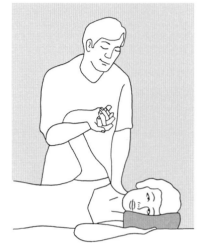

Stretching the Neck in the Side-Lying Position

Try different handholds to see if you can apply a gentle stretch to the shoulder and neck muscles in the side-lying position. Which method suits you best, standing at the head of the couch and gently depressing the client's shoulder or hooking your arm in theirs to depress the shoulder that way?

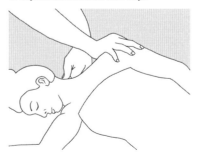

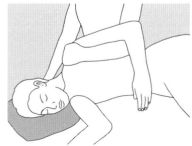

Forearm Massage in the Side-Lying Position

In Tip 8 (pp. 70–73) you saw how changing the position of the shoulder in the prone position facilitated greater access to trapezius. Changing the position of the client entirely, from prone to three-quarter lying, is another way to help you access these tissues.

Sitting or kneeling at the head of the treatment couch, use your forearm to gently work into the tissues once you have warmed them up.

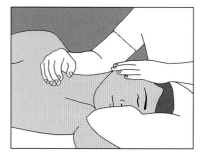

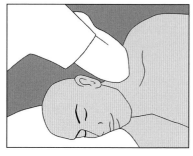

Be careful to keep your pressure light as you move over the transverse processes of the cervical vertebrae as too much pressure could cause bruising and discomfort. Deeper pressure can be used in the fleshy belly of the upper fibers of trapezius.

Tip 12: Tips for Treating the Neck with Your Client Seated

Abduction of the Arm in Seated Position

Practice palpating the upper part of trapezius with your client in a seated position. How do the tissues feel? Are they soft and malleable or dense and stiff?

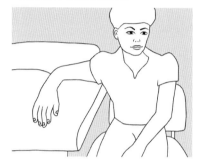

Next, find a way to passively abduct the shoulder of your client, perhaps using pillows. By placing the arm into passive abduction, there is less tension on the upper part of trapezius and you have the advantage of being able to access underlying tissues more easily. In this altered position, palpate the upper fibers of trapezius again. How do the tissues feel now, is there a difference?

Gripping Trapezius with and without Rotation

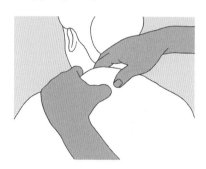

Another technique with your client seated, with or without passive arm abduction, is to gently grip the tissues of trapezius. This is not always possible, for, as you know, some clients have strong, dense tissues which are stiff and difficult to grip. However, sometimes simple gripping is all that is required to facilitate a reduction in tension.

An additional technique is to maintain a grip and to ask your client to gently turn their head away from you, bringing about a soft tissue stretch.

Transverse Strokes

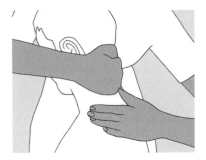

Gently stroking the tissues transversely away from the spine is soothing but requires you to support the client's head as shown, and not all clients feel comfortable in this position. In the sitting position, the muscles of the neck are active as they try to support the head, so this is not the most effective treatment position for reducing tension here. It is, however, useful when a client is unable, or does not wish, to lie on a couch to receive treatment.

Pressing into the Occiput

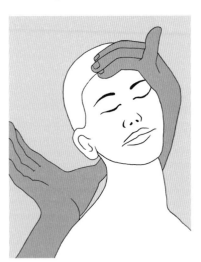

This can be helpful for applying gentle pressure to the suboccipital muscles. Taking the head gently back into extension helps shorten the neck extensor muscles, facilitating greater access to deeper structures.

Linked Fingers to "Pull Off" Soft Tissues

Standing behind your subject, link your fingers, squeezing the soft tissues toward you. Keep your pressure light to avoid squashing tissues forcibly against the transverse processes of cervical vertebrae.

Alternatively, gently grip and draw the tissues toward you.

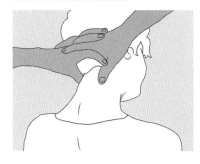

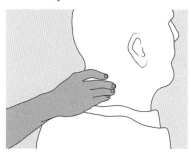

Use this chart and tick the boxes when you have practiced these seven techniques on three different clients.

Technique		1	2	3
1. Seated (without arm abduction)				
2. Seated with arm in abduction	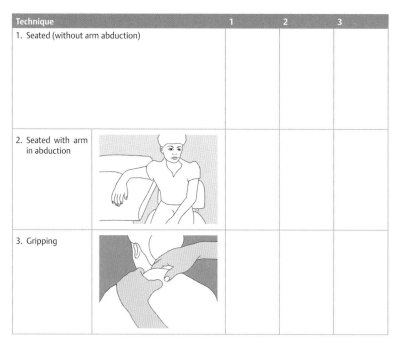			
3. Gripping				

Technique		1	2	3
4. Gripping with active rotation				
5. Transverse strokes				
6. Gentle pressures to occiput				
7. Gentle gripping to back of neck				

Tip 13: Treating Suboccipitals

In Chapter 1, the importance of the small occipital muscles was described in Tip 19 (p. 38), and Tip 20 (p. 39) covered how to palpate them. Here you will find some tips on ways you might treat these muscles, using various different treatment positions.

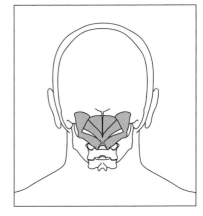

Prone

In the prone position, you can use your fingertips to gently massage the suboccipital area as you stand at the head of the couch or you can simply rest your fingertips against the base of the skull and allow the gentlest of fingertip pressure to stimulate a decrease in tension. Sometimes, using your thumbs to gently press into the muscles on one side of the neck and then to gently push the skin from the occiput, down toward the base of the neck and toward the shoulders can be very soothing. Fingers or thumbs can be reinforced, but often only very light touch is needed as you move from the hairline, down toward the lower cervical vertebrae.

TIP: As you practice either of these techniques— resting your fingertips or pushing the skin—ask yourself whether both left and right sides of the occipital region feel the same. If one feels different, in what way is it different? Is it more firm to palpate? More pliable? Less pliable? Do the tissues seem to move in the same manner as on the opposite side of the occiput? Can you identify any localized trigger points or do you feel that this region of the neck is too dense for you to identify trigger points through palpation?

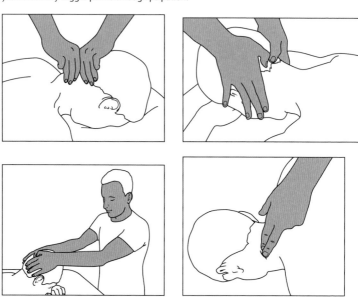

Supine

In the supine position, posterior neck muscles are relaxed, and palpation can sometimes be easier than when the client is prone. Working with a client supine, you have the opportunity to assess the suboccipital region for tenderness and trigger points and to use the weight of the client's head to assist in the treatment.

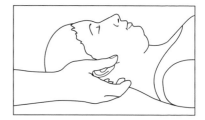

For example, consider the following steps:

STEP 1 Just as when working with your client prone, sit for a while with your fingers at the base of their skull. See if you can identify any differences between the left and the right sides of the occipital bone where trapezius inserts. Is one side more tender than the other? Move your fingertips off the bone and onto soft tissue, right at the base of the skull, the topmost part of the neck. How do the tissues feel? Experiment with the placement of your fingers and identify which is most comfortable for you when you remain in the same position for a few moments. Where do you need to rest your elbows in order to be comfortable? Does it make a difference how high or how low you position your treatment couch? Do you feel more comfortable sitting, kneeling, or squatting?

STEP 2 Once you are comfortable, flex your metacarpophalangeal joints as shown here, taking the weight of the client's head onto your fingers, and let the head gently roll from side to

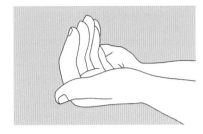

side. Do not force any movements; instead, simply allow the client's head to move onto or off your fingertips. Does the head roll easily both to the left and to the right or does it get "stuck" anywhere? How does this gentle palpation with rocking feel for your client? How does your own body feel when you provide treatment in this position? Are you comfortable or do you start to get backache? It is important to safeguard your posture, and you may find that it takes a while to find the position that is comfortable for both your back and for your hands.

Summary of questions to ask when treating suboccipital muscles in the supine position

Do both left and right suboccipitals feel the same?

If they feel different to you, in what way do they feel different? Is there an increase/decrease in tone on one side?

Does the client report one side as being more tender than the other?

Where do you need to rest your elbows, on or off the couch?

Do you feel more comfortable sitting, kneeling, or squatting?

Does it make a difference if you raise/lower your treatment couch?

Side-Lying Position

Another way to treat the suboccipital area is with your client in the side-lying position. Here you can gently run your thumb from the base of the neck toward the occiput, dragging the skin gently in a cephalic direction and stopping when you reach the occipital bone. This is useful as it enables you to really focus on the suboccipital muscles on one side of the neck.

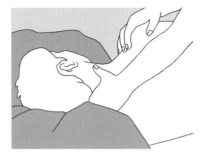

Experimenting with (or without) a pillow means you can practice this gentle stripping motion with the tissues of the posterior neck shortened (usually with a pillow) or lengthened and under a little tension (usually without a pillow).

The advantage of not using a pillow is that you can experiment with varying degrees of head flexion/extension, asking your client to perform a nodding motion.

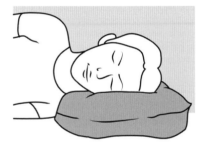

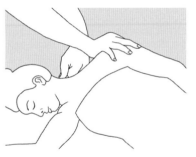

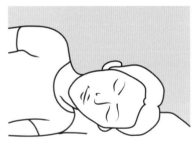

You can also practice changing the position of the client's arm. How does changing the position of the client's arm affect both you and your client?

Passively abducting the arm shortens the tissues spanning the arm and shoulder and with them slackened, you can palpate to deeper structures. Alternatively, with the arm resting against the client's body, the tissues on the lateral side of the neck are tensioned, especially if you apply a little depression to the shoulder. Notice what happens when your client gently nods their head in this side-lying position as you palpate the scalenes on one side of their neck. Sometimes you can facilitate relief simply by applying fingertip pressure as the client performs this rhythmic nodding movement.

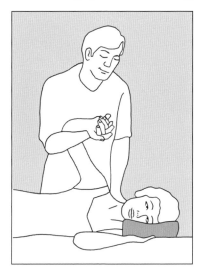

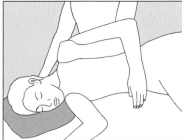

Seated

With your client seated, you can allow their head to fall gently back onto your thumbs and can thus apply gentle pressure to one side of the occipital region at a time with relative ease to yourself. You will find that you need to support the client's forehead as shown. While we need to guard against injury to our thumbs as therapists, this technique does not require deep pressure nor does it require you to rotate your thumb. Simply allow the suboccipital tissues to rest gently on your thumb for about 5 to 10 seconds before moving your thumb to a new position.

Ohashi (1977) suggests using a headband to help as you press your thumbs gently into the soft tissues of the occipital region. This area can be sore for many clients, so avoid holding any point for too long and avoid overworking the area in general.

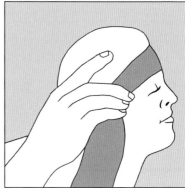

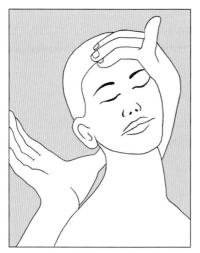

Tip 14: Understanding Levator Scapulae

The levator scapulae is an interesting muscle. It can be felt as a strap-like band running up the back of the neck on either side, deep to trapezius. Originating on the transverse processes of the upper three or four cervical vertebrae and inserting into the superior angle of the scapulae, when it is "tight" it is palpable as a twangy band, about 2 cm in width. Often, palpation and compression of this muscle elicits feelings of tenderness and relief simultaneously. As a result, it is tempting to massage this area deeply in an attempt to help stretch the muscle and not least because clients enjoy the sensation of relief such deep massage brings about. However, if we stop for a moment to consider the anatomy and function of the levator scapulae, it becomes obvious that our attempts to lengthen this muscle may not be advantageous.

The levator scapulae is very much like the reigns of a horse, and it often works to reign in the head, helping to reposition the head over the thorax where it belongs, and where tension on supportive tissues is lessened. Often, when a client presents with a forward-head posture, craning their head as if hurrying, the levator scapulae is forced to adopt a lengthened position. Tension in the muscle increases as it works *isometrically* to maintain head position, *eccentrically* as the head falls forward, and *concentrically* in an attempt to bring the head back over the body. It is not surprising that people with a forward-head posture often complain of neck pain.

While deep tissue massage and stretching are enjoyable to receive, and certainly help in reducing muscular tension, one of the long-term goals for clients with forward-head posture is to help them to correct this posture and to shorten the levator scapulae. For ideas on how clients can be helped to learn to do this for themselves, please see Chapter 3, Tip 7: Neck Retractions (pp. 131–133).

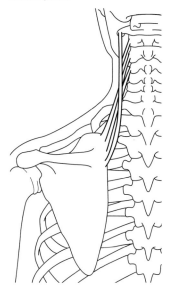

Tip 15: Addressing Trigger Points in the Levator Scapulae

A useful technique for addressing pain and decreasing muscle tension in the neck is to palpate the levator scapulae for trigger points and to try to reduce these. Sometimes this is achieved to great satisfaction if you position your client on their side and apply gentle pressure at a 90-degree angle onto the trigger point.

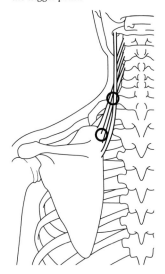

Trigger points in the levator scapulae may also be addressed with your client prone or seated and it is worth experimenting with each to see which position works best for you.

STEP 1 With your client in the chosen treatment position, start by warming up the area.

STEP 2 Using light strokes to begin, cover the area slowly, and consistently, using your fingertips to search for trigger spots. If after stroking the whole region you have not located any

trigger points, repeat the process with slightly firmer strokes, palpating into a deeper layer of tissue. Remember to work *slowly*. Triggers will be discovered as palpable, tender points that often run in bands. They are often located close to where the elevator scapulae inserts onto the superior angle of the scapula.

STEP 3 If you find a trigger point, rest your thumb or finger gently on the point and wait. Your client may feel some tenderness but should be able to tolerate your pressure without experiencing any pain. Within about 60 seconds, you should feel a reduction in tension in this localized point and your client should report a decrease in tenderness. Soothe the area with massage before seeking out and treating another spot in the same manner.

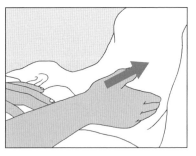

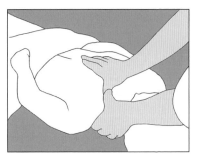

TIP: It sometimes helps to encourage the client to imagine the tenderness simply melting away. Sometimes, with a verbal prompt such as this, both you and the client perceive this decrease in tone in the muscle.

Question: How long should I hold the trigger point for?

Hold the point until there is a decrease in tenderness. Usually this occurs within about 10 to 12 seconds but varies between individuals. If the trigger point is chronic, it may take longer to "release," but this is not always the case. Sometimes, the relief the client experiences simply from the pressure of gentle palpation at that particular point is so great that the decrease in muscle tone is apparent within seconds. At other times, you may find that you are holding a point for around 60 seconds and that any decrease in tone is very minor. The trick is not to try and force the release of a point. Again, working to the less-is-more principle, several attempts using light touch can be more effective than trying to physically *push* a point away with brute force!

Many people find that a gentle neck stretch following the release of trigger points helps "reset" the muscle to its original length. This could be an active stretch or a passive stretch. Alternatively, simply taking the head through some of the cervical ranges of movement can be a nice way to finish a trigger point session.

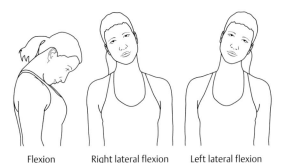

Flexion   Right lateral flexion   Left lateral flexion

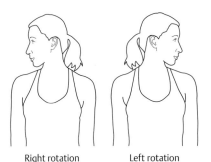

Right rotation   Left rotation

Tip 16: Positional Release for the Levator Scapulae

If you discover tender spots in the levator scapulae, one way to address these is to use a technique known as positional release or strain–counterstrain developed by Lawrence Jones, a doctor of osteopathy. This technique involves repositioning your client so that their discomfort feels eased. You first need to identify the tender spot and then to passively slacken the soft tissues associated with this spot. In the case of the levator scapulae, this means taking the client's head and neck into gentle lateral flexion on the side of the tenderness. With the neck laterally flexed and the shoulder passively elevated, the fibers of the levator scapulae are in a shortened position. There are many ways to do this, and it is likely that you will need to use different treatment positions for different clients. Once in the treatment position—seated, supine, or side lying—you need to experiment to find the position in which your client feels *most* ease from their discomfort.

You can try this technique for yourself by following these very basic steps:

STEP 1 With your client seated, find a comfortable position in which to passively elevate the scapula. This could be with your client seated next to a couch, their arm supported on the couch, or they could rest their arm over your thigh if you felt that that was appropriate for them. In this position, palpate for tender spots in the levator scapulae. Rest your finger on a spot when you find one. If you are able to identify more than one spot, running in a band, choose the point in the middle.

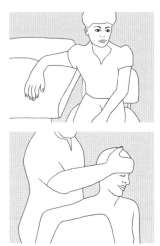

STEP 2 Find the position of ease. Help place the levator scapulae into a passively shortened position by easing the client's head into lateral flexion, or extension, or rotation, or a combination of these movements. The client should report a 70% reduction in discomfort in the tender spot you are palpating once in the position of ease.

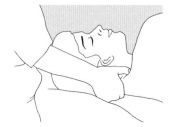

You may find this is easier to facilitate with the client in the side-lying position, which has the advantage of prompting greater relaxation and a reduction in muscle tone, whereas when a client is seated, the muscles of neck extension are active in order to support the weight of the head.

STEP 3 Hold this position for 90 seconds while continuing to palpate the tender spot, and then gently return the client's head to the neutral position. In neutral, recheck the tender spot. There should be less discomfort on palpation.

For an interesting discussion on this topic, see Fallon and Walsh (2012).

Question: Are the tender spots that respond to *strain–counterstrain* the same as trigger points?

No. They are localized like trigger points, about 1 cm in diameter, and represent either neuromuscular or musculoskeletal dysfunction, but they do not respond to techniques such as soft tissue release (STR; described in the next tip) or to spray-and-stretch techniques. Nor do they respond to injections the way trigger points do.

Tip 17: Soft Tissue Release to Trapezius/Levator Scapulae

Another way to help decrease tone and stretch soft tissues in the posterior neck region is to use STR. This pin-and-stretch technique is helpful for alleviating the discomfort of trigger points. It is a relatively safe form of neck stretching because when STR is applied to the neck, it is the client who is in charge of how far they choose to stretch, not the therapist.

This tip explains how to apply STR to both the trapezius and the levator scapulae. In practice, these two muscles cannot be separated anatomically for the purposes of treatment, due to their fascial connections. Yet like other techniques (such as stretches and positional release technique), it is possible to place the focus of the technique more on one muscle than the other, bearing in mind that both will be affected, one to a lesser degree and one to a greater degree.

Focusing STR to Trapezius

STEP 1 Massage the upper back and neck to warm and soothe the tissues.

STEP 2 Apply gentle pressure to the belly of the upper fibers of trapezius, avoiding bony points such as the clavicle and acromion process.

You can apply pressure using your thumb, finger, reinforced fingers, or, with caution, your elbow. In the illustration below, the therapist is using her forearm, attempting to gently compress the tissues, forming a "lock." She is standing behind the client using her right arm, but she could have chosen to stand to the side of the client and use her left arm.

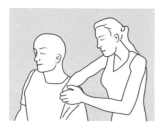

STEP 3 While maintaining gentle pressure, ask your client to slowly take their head away from you. They should experience a stretch to the soft tissues to the side of their neck. Hold the position for about 10 seconds, then release your lock and ask your client to return their head to neutral. Repeat two more times on this spot, or choose a different spot on which to work.

STR should be comfortable and pain free. There is sometimes slight tenderness, but this should be tolerable. If the client experiences pain, you should stop. Also, be cautious in using this technique on clients who have had problems such as lumbar herniations. Forces even from gentle compression of the trapezius (or the levator scapulae) are transmitted to the spine and could aggravate a preexisting spinal condition.

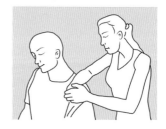

Focusing STR to the Levator Scapulae

Here you will need to change the position of your lock so that you are more directly over this muscle. Also, the direction in which the client needs to stretch is different.

STEP 1 As for the upper fibers of trapezius, locate an area of soft tissue and apply a gentle lock. Here the therapist has chosen to use her elbow to fix the tissues. Remember, using an elbow does not necessitate more force; it is simply a different "tool" with which to apply the gentle "lock."

STEP 2 While maintaining the lock, ask the client to rotate their head away from you about 45 degrees and then to look to the floor. They will experience a stretch of the posterolateral side of the neck. Soothe the area with general massage and then repeat STR on this same side, moving to a slightly different spot, or apply the stretch to the opposite side of the neck. Experiment with placing your lock in different positions on the neck and get feedback as to which head and neck movement the client needs to perform in order to experience the best sense of stretch and release.

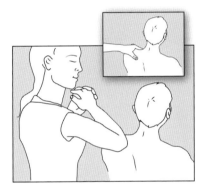

Question: What if my client experiences referred sensations?

This technique should feel comfortable to receive and the client should experience a sense of relief following it. However, it is common for clients to report referred symptoms in other parts of their body such as the head, face, arm, and chest. This is normal when there are trigger points present and your pressure is directly over a trigger point. The technique should never cause pain, and if your client reports pain, you should stop.

For more information on this technique, see Johnson (2009).

Tip 18: **Treating Scalenes**

In *The Trigger Point Therapy Workbook* (Davies, 2004), the author describes how trigger points located within the scalene muscles can refer pain to other parts of the body such as the arm, forearm, thumb, upper chest, and scapula. To alleviate such discomfort, apply STR, using the steps described in the figure below.

The scalene muscles

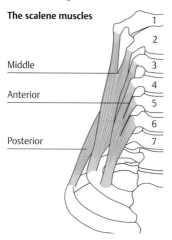

Middle

Anterior

Posterior

1
2
3
4
5
6
7

STEP 2 Once you are sure you have located a scalene, use the pads of your fingers to apply *gentle* pressure to the muscle superior to the clavicle.

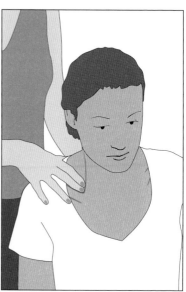

STEP 1 Remind yourself about the anatomy of scalenes and observe your client to see whether the scalenes on one side of the neck are more prominent at rest. Following the steps in Chapter 1, Tip 14 (p. 33), locate scalenes on your subject.

STEP 3 Maintaining this gentle pressure, ask your client to turn their head away from your finger. Your subject should experience a mild stretch on the anterolateral side of their neck as they do this, releasing tension here. After a few seconds, ask them to return their head to the start position (neutral) and repeat once more.

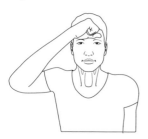

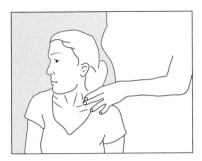

Palpate the scalenes on the opposite side of the neck. How does the tension in this side compare with the tension in the muscles you have just treated? Is it increased or decreased? Apply STR to the opposite side of the neck. Check whether the application of this technique has increased the range of movement in your client's neck and/or decreased their discomfort.

Tip 19: **Treating Sternocleidomastoid**

Sternocleidomastoid may become hypertonic in clients with poor posture or following whiplash injuries. It may be strained during sporting activities and activities such as overhead weightlifting. As it becomes active during deep inspiration, when lung volume reaches about 75%, and when a sudden intake of breath is required, it can sometimes be seen in singers and public speakers and is an important muscle of respiration for people engaged in heavy physical activity. Many clients do not realize they have tension in their sternocleidomastoid muscle until they receive gentle palpation and massage.

Although some therapists choose to massage the length of this muscle, it is wise to work with sensitivity and caution due to the proximity of important structures on the anterior of the neck.

One way to treat sternocleidomastoid is to massage the area and then to apply a gentle stretch, placing one hand on the sternum, and applying slight traction with the other, at the side of the head. You can modify this stretch by gently rotating the head to one side and repositioning your hands.

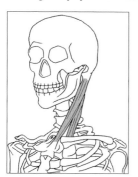
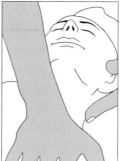
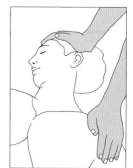

TIP: Pressure on the belly of the muscle can stimulate a cough reflex and can make some clients feel uncomfortable, especially if both the left and the right sides of the neck were massaged at the same time. For this reason, it is often more effective to restrict your treatment to gentle circling of the origins (sternum and clavicle) and insertion (mastoid process) of the muscle.

For an interesting article on the activity patterns of sternocleidomastoid and latissimus dorsi in classical singers, see Watson et al (2012). Also, Min et al (2010) provide a case study of a subject with auricular pain that was discovered to be derived from trigger points in sternocleidomastoid.

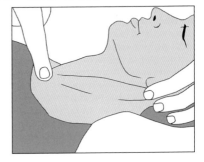

Tip 20: Muscle Energy Technique to the Neck

Muscle energy technique (MET) is a form of stretching and strengthening. It has many applications and many variations and is useful when treating people with neck conditions. Included here are descriptions of two ways (bilateral and unilateral) in which you can use MET to help stretch muscles of the neck, specifically the muscles responsible for shoulder elevation and lateral flexion of the neck. Note that while the protocol described here uses a 10-second contraction and 10% of the client's force, this is only one method of applying MET, and one of the simplest.

There are many variations of the technique and you are likely to come across therapists who use MET slightly differently. If you are new to this technique, try it and be prepared to modify it to suit your needs and those of your clients.

As MET requires the client to perform an isometric contraction, it should only be used on clients for whom it is safe. An example of a client for whom it may not be safe would be someone with unmedicated high blood pressure, as an increase in muscle tone increases blood pressure.

Supine, Bilaterally

Use this method of application if your client is comfortable having both of their shoulders depressed at the same time.

STEP 1 With your client comfortably positioned in the supine position, gently depress their shoulders, applying pressure caudally.

STEP 2 Ask your client to shrug their shoulders, using about 10% of their force. Do not allow their shoulders to elevate. However, be wary of pushing their shoulders down. *You* are resisting the force provided by the client; the client should not be trying to resist you.

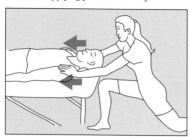

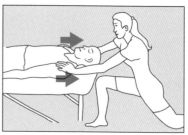

STEP 3 After about 10 seconds, ask your client to relax, and then slowly depress their shoulders a little more. Hold them in this new, depressed position. Repeat once more if your client is willing.

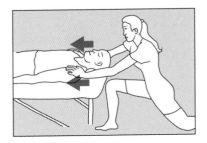

TIP: Instead of depressing the shoulders a second time, once your client has stopped shrugging, ask them to remain in the same position but to try and reach their hands toward their toes, depressing their own shoulders. This engages the lower fibers of trapezius as well as other muscles and can be helpful in decreasing tone in the upper fibers of this muscle.

The advantage of this method is that it saves time (you can stretch both sides of the neck at once) and it can be useful when stretching the neck muscles of clients who are hypermobile and for whom the supine unilateral stretch is not appropriate. The disadvantage is that it cannot be used with clients who have an acute shoulder injury such as supraspinatus tendonitis, acromioclavicular joint injuries, injury to the lateral third of the clavicle, or subdeltoid bursitis, as it does require some pressure, albeit gentle, to be applied to the head of the humerus.

Supine, Unilaterally

Use this method of application if your client has a shoulder problem and you think bilateral MET may aggravate this. Or simply use it as an alternative to depressing the shoulders bilaterally.

STEP 1 With your client comfortably positioned in the supine position, place one hand on their shoulder and another on the side of their face. Gently apply pressure, taking their head into lateral flexion.

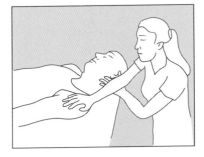

STEP 2 Keeping your hands here, the head and shoulder fixed, ask your client to try to bring their head back to a neutral position while shrugging their shoulder, using about 10% of their force. You can see that this engages the lateral flexors of the neck. Again, be wary of pushing your client's head and shoulder apart: *You* should be resisting the force provided by your client; your client should not be trying to resist you.

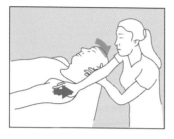

STEP 3 After about 10 seconds, ask your client to relax, and then slowly take the neck a little more into lateral flexion.

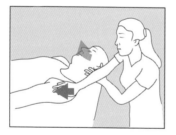

Hold the head in this new position, encouraging your client to breathe normally and relax. If a client has a very stiff neck, with a decreased range of lateral flexion, you may wish to perform this again on the same side. However, the neck does not require a great deal of gross lateral flexion, so it is sometimes better to err on the side of caution and apply other techniques to help loosen stiffness and increase range of movement than to attempt to stretch the neck again using MET. Repeat on the other side of the neck.

The advantage of this method is that it can be used to help stretch the neck of a client who cannot receive MET bilaterally. The disadvantages are that it can be too severe for some clients and care must be taken not to overstretch the tissues. For this reason, it is not appropriate for clients who are hypermobile, who already have a good range of movement into lateral flexion of their neck. Another disadvantage is that when the neck is taken into lateral flexion, muscles are shortened on one side of the neck, and they risk cramping.

Tip 21: Taping the Neck

This chapter ends with a tip about tape. It is a tip designed to raise questions and to stimulate your thinking!

The use of tape to help improve muscle function is not new but is becoming increasingly popular due to new versions of tape that are now available to therapists. If you intend to use tape with the intention of helping a client to improve function or to decrease pain in their neck, you should consider undertaking special training. However, you should also bear in mind that results for the use of tape are mixed. While certain types of tape are valuable in restricting movement, there is less evidence for the use of tape to decrease pain and enhance movement. For this reason, it is difficult to describe a specific protocol for the use of tape when treating clients with neck conditions.

The starting point when considering the use of tape as a therapeutic modality should be to ask yourself for what purpose is it being used. What are your therapeutic goals?

Examples of therapeutic goals are the following:

- To decrease pain.
- To decrease discomfort.
- To decrease stiffness.
- To decrease muscle tone.
- To increase muscle tone.
- To improve range of movement.
- To improve function (as in activities of daily living or sporting function).
- To help correct postural imbalance.

Ask yourself next whether there are other interventions that would be as good as, or better than, the application of tape.

A common condition you may already have come across is that of a forward-head posture, with clients complaining of pain and soreness in their neck and shoulders as a result of muscle imbalance. It seems reasonable to assume that tape could be used to help the client maintain a better head and neck posture if the tape were applied in such a way as to temporarily correct posture and discourage the "chin" poke position many people fall into. In this example, tape could be applied to the upper trapezius in such a manner that when the client's posture falters, and they start craning forward, the tape is tensioned and they are alerted to correct their posture. However, it needs to be remembered that tape is thought to stimulate mechanoreceptors and in doing so is likely to increase tone in muscles. Is this what you would want to achieve in the upper fibers of the trapezius in a client with poor posture?

Some tape manufacturers claim that their tape can be used to decrease muscle tone if it is applied in a particular manner. If you wanted to decrease tone in the upper fibers of the trapezius, for example, would using tape be your best treatment approach or could you use another treatment modality to achieve this goal?

Chapter III

Neck Aftercare

Chapter 3 **Neck Aftercare**

It can be a struggle sometimes to know what to say to a client who is in pain with a recent neck injury or who has been suffering with a neck problem for many months or years. Often clients want a "quick fix" or they are fearful of reinjury and scared to move their neck at all. Sometimes a person is simply worn down by the constant discomfort of a chronic neck condition or with having to cope with a neck condition that flares up unexpectedly.

The 11 *tips* in this chapter are all about the kinds of information you can give to your clients to help them to manage their neck conditions. This includes information you can provide to help explain their condition and how best to recover from neck problems, advise on safe stretches, and simple exercises they can perform, as well as a few tricks you may not have come across. The chapter begins with tips about how we can help educate, advise, and reassure clients by throwing light on neck care facts which you, as a therapist, may take for granted, but which clients may not be aware of.

As therapists, it is probable that we are more informed about the body than most of our clients, and an important part of our role is to help educate people as to how they can prevent, manage, and resolve their symptoms. Of course, there are many clients with a high level of understanding about anatomy and physiology, and about injury and rehabilitation, especially if they are keen on being able to take part in a regular physical activity and want to lessen their chances of injury. However, even when a client exercises regularly and is fairly well informed, this does not mean that they have the same knowledge and appreciation about their bodies as we therapists do. It is common for clients to use the internet to seek solutions to their neck problems. The internet is not only a fantastic source for sharing knowledge, but also contains much misinformation. We have an ideal opportunity to help clients care for their necks and manage their neck complaints in a safe and appropriate way.

Tip 1: **Playing Sherlock**

One of the reasons why neck problems persist can be because a client continues to do something that aggravates their symptoms. Aggravating and easing factors are usually identified during the initial assessment and the information is used to help identify the condition the client is suffering from. The identification of aggravating factors is included here, as part of aftercare, because it often requires the client to take concerted action, outside of the therapy clinic, in order to determine what these aggravating factors are. Often a client can tell you immediately which movements, activities, or conditions give rise to more discomfort, pain, or a "flare up" of their neck problem, but in some cases they cannot. Sometimes, an aggravating factor is an activity that is so commonplace that the client fails to recognize it as an aggravating factor at all. The longer a person has been doing an activity, and the more commonplace it is for them, the less likely they are to consider it an aggravating factor. This is where we, as therapists, can help by asking open-ended questions that may prompt awareness.

Further, the aggravating factor does not necessarily need to involve movement. A task that involves a person to keep his/her neck in a static position for a long period of time can also be problematic. Examples of when the head and neck are held static or almost static are reading, using a microscope, bird-watching, concentrating on close-work hobbies such as needlecraft, sitting at a desk using a laptop or computer, and watching television.

Question: What if my client cannot identify any aggravating factors?

A useful tip here is to suggest that your client keep an activity diary for 7 days, for a period of time that represents their normal routine. When the client returns for another appointment with you, ask them what it was they were doing when their symptom came on, and try to get as specific as possible. Were they moving or staying still? If they were moving, what were they doing? Can they remember which movement they made? Did it involve their neck only or did it involve their arms or shoulders too? Were they lifting or carrying anything, for example? Was it a whole body activity? Were they engaged in sport or exercise? If they told you, for example, that it came on when they were swimming, what stroke were they doing? A common example of a stroke that aggravates neck pain in some people is when the client does breaststroke while keeping their head above the water, their neck in extension. If the activity involved moving only their head, what did they do? Ask them in layperson's terms whether they looked down (flexion), up to the ceiling (extension), over one shoulder (rotation), etc. Was it a combination of movements? If the client was in a static position when the symptom came on, what were they doing? Where they standing, sitting, crouching, or lying? If they were lying, in which position? On their back, side, or stomach? If the symptom came on when they were lying on their stomach with their head turned to the right, for example, does the symptom also come on when they rest prone with their head to the left? If they were sitting, what were they doing? Were they reading? Watching television? Did they fall asleep? If they fell asleep and woke up with neck pain, where were their head and neck when they woke up? Had the head dropped forward or to one side?

Where a symptom develops from a static posture, you will need to help the client identify whether it is the posture itself that aggravates the symptom or whether the symptom is duration-dependent. For example, if a person's pain comes on when they remain static in order to read, for how long can they read (remain in this posture) before the symptom develops?

Once you have specific information concerning aggravating factors, you are a short step away from providing the client with preventative advice.

Question: Do clients really need help identifying aggravating factors?

It may seem obvious that if a symptom develops after retaining a static posture for 40 minutes, for example, the solution is simply to avoid this position for more than, say, 30 minutes. Yet we all fall victim to these kinds of habits and having someone point out that we are sitting too long, for example, is a good thing. You have probably come across plenty of clients who will tell you, "Yeah, I know, you're right, it's just that when I'm into it I can't seem to stop," or "I forgot the time." Maybe a solution would be to print a line of copy in books which says, "Stop, you have read 100 pages; do you need to take a break?" (By the way, if you are reading this book cover to cover, stop; you have read 117 pages.)

Useful Exploratory Questions to Help Identify Aggravating Factors

Use these questions to prompt your own thinking and to help you when questioning clients in order to try and identify aggravating factors which you can then eliminate or reduce. These are by no means exhaustive, and are in no particular order, but will hopefully provide a jumping-off point for further investigation.

When you noticed your symptom:

Were you moving or staying still?

If you were moving, what were you doing?

Can you remember which movement you made? Did it involve your neck only or did it involve you arms or shoulders too?

Were you lifting or carrying anything?

Were you shrugging your shoulders?

Where were your arms? Were they hanging loose by your sides, supported on a chair, or in some other position?

Did you notice your symptom following a whole body activity such as sport or exercise? If so, what were you doing and which part of the activity aggravated the symptom? For example, if you were swimming, what stroke were you doing?

If you moved only your head before the symptom came on, what did you do? Did you look down (flexion), up to the ceiling (extension), over one shoulder (rotation), or was it some other movement? Can you show me what you did?

If you were in a static position when the symptom came on, what were you doing? Where you standing, sitting, crouching, or lying?

If you were lying, in which position? On your back, side, or stomach? In which position were your head and neck? Can you show me?

If you were sitting, what were you doing? How were you sitting? Upright, or slumped, on a chair or on a sofa, at work, the cinema, in a cafe, or at home? Can you show me how you were sitting?

Were you reading, watching television, or doing a craft activity? Can you show me the position you were in while doing this activity?

Did you fall asleep sitting? Where were your head and neck when you woke up? Had the head dropped forward or to one side?

For how long can you remain in this static posture before the symptom develops?

Question: Why do we need to bother being so "specific" in trying to identify aggravating factors?

First, aggravating factors help us clinicians to determine the condition we are dealing with. Secondly, once we know what aggravates a person's symptoms, we can help them to find ways to eliminate or avoid these things.

Example of How Getting Specific Information Can Help Identify Aggravating Factors

A client comes to you with a recurring neck problem and tells you they cannot identify anything that makes it worse. As part of your home care advice, you suggest that they keep a 7-day diary and when they return a week later they tell you that they still cannot identify what is aggravating their pain, only that "It came on when I went to see my neighbor." You ask what they were doing and they reply, "I wasn't doing anything different. It was a normal day." Your task is to be the Sherlock Holmes of therapists, to discover what was different that particular day, that particular occasion. Has visiting their neighbor ever triggered this symptom before? What were they doing during the visit? Does the trigger have to do with how they sit or stand at a neighbor's house? You ask the client to tell you exactly what they did ("Just the usual. We had coffee."). So you ask, "Was anything different that day at all?" What would you think if they then said, "Nothing. Only I didn't have my scarf that day"?

"Do you usually wear a scarf?" you ask. They tell you that they always wear a scarf and when you ask, "Why?" they say, "I don't know. I just feel better with it on."

"So what happened when you visited your neighbor that day when you didn't have a scarf on?"

"Nothing, but my neck started hurting."

"What were you doing?"

"Drinking coffee."

Then the client remembers, "It was cold."

So now you are faced with an opportunity: was the symptom brought on by holding a particular posture to drink coffee, retaining this posture for a long period of time, sitting to drink coffee in a cold environment, or was it something altogether different that also happened while at the neighbor's house that triggered the neck pain? Later the client says, "Come to think of it, I think the cold does make it worse." You ask them to explain. "When I go to the cinema I can't sit in an aisle seat because if there's a draft my neck hurts." Then they remember that when they sat in a restaurant one time under some air conditioning vent, they had neck pain the following day.

You can see that from the information generated in this particular example, you are starting to build up a picture of causal factors and might surmise that the client has a neck condition aggravated by cold temperatures. This kind of questioning and the responses the client gives help your client realize just how important it is for them to keep their neck warm.

Although identification of aggravating factors is part of your initial assessment, you can see now how encouraging a client to identify aggravating factors themselves is key to successful intervention.

Identifying Obsolete Exercises

A client may be reluctant to consider that an exercise they have been doing regularly could be an aggravating factor, especially if it was an activity which they took up initially to help overcome a problem, and which seemed to help alleviate the problem at the time.

Example 1: A client may have once been advised to do neck "rolls," circumducting their head which at the time alleviated their symptoms. Perhaps they were retaining a static posture for long periods of time and neck rolls were a way of alleviating tension in the muscles of the neck and shoulders?

Perhaps they had a stiff neck and a reduced range of movement (ROM) and so neck rolls were given as a means of encouraging the client to move through, and improve, all ranges. Three years later, performing end-of-range neck rolls every hour while sitting at their desk may not be appropriate.

Example 2: A client may have been told as a child that doing headstands is good for core stability and would help keep their neck strong. Years later, trying to do headstands as part of a neck-strengthening regime following a whiplash accident is probably not advisable.

Clients sometimes continue to perform exercises prophylactically, believing these to likely prevent their symptoms from returning. Whilst some neck exercises are useful to perform regularly, most are prescribed to help manage a specific condition, at a specific point in time in the course of a person's recovery. Many clients stick to old regimes believing these to be helpful when these may at best be ineffective now, or at worst are aggravating a condition. One of your tasks is to help identify where a client is performing an exercise that has long since become obsolete for the client's needs, and to help educate them in this.

Tip 2: Acute versus Chronic – Basic Advice

Advice for Clients with either Acute or Chronic Neck Pain

- Reassure your client that X-rays and MRI scans often reveal degenerative changes in the cervical vertebrae. It would be wrong to assume that a neck problem is due solely to these changes. Many people whose necks show signs of degeneration are problem free and experience no pain and no stiffness. Degenerative change is normal and happens to us all as we age.
- Reassure your client by telling them that the neck often makes a creaking sound known as "crepitus." This does not necessarily mean there is anything wrong.

- Reassure your client that there is much that can be done to help them, and many different interventions they can try. As a therapist, consider the main problem—is it pain, stiffness, impairment of function, etc.—and brainstorm all of the things you know are useful in addressing each of these.
- Ask your client to consider the general advice provided here as well as the advice on staying active.

Advice for a Client with Acute Neck Pain

- Most acute neck pain resolves at best within a few days, at worst within a few weeks.
- The sooner you return to normal daily activities, the sooner you are likely to get better.
- The sooner you are able to move your neck, the sooner you are likely to get better.
- People who avoid moving their neck and avoid returning to their daily activities are at greater risk of suffering chronic neck pain and report coping less well with their pain.
- People who start moving and who try to return to normal are likely to recover quickly and to cope best with neck pain.

- Modify your activities to start with.
- When we damage the outside of our bodies, we see evidence of damage—a wound, bruise, scab, or scar. When we damage the insides of our body, we cannot see the damage. The body needs time to heal on the inside just as on the outside, with blood vessels, muscles, tendons and ligaments, and, in some cases, fractures repairing themselves, and nerve inflammations settling down. Pain often resolves before the healing process is complete, so most of the time we simply need to be patient.
- Most causes of neck pain are not serious.

Advice for a Client with Chronic Neck Pain

- For clients who suffer isolated episodes of pain, try to discover if there is a trig-

ger. Encourage your client to try and pinpoint what brought on their pain. If necessary, review Tip 1 in this chapter, to see if you can identify aggravating factors and remove or eliminate these.

- If the pain is due to an underlying condition such as degenerative changes in cervical vertebrae, remind your client that between episodes they often experience weeks or even months when they are pain free or have much reduced levels of pain.

- If you feel it is appropriate, ask your client to consider pain medication as one way of managing if their pain is constant. Medication may not need to be taken all of the time but can be a useful way of helping clients to cope.

- For clients suffering chronic pain, suggest they consider trying to pace their activities, reducing the duration or intensity of what they do. For example, make several shopping trips, carrying lighter shopping each time.

- Suggest a client to consider attending a pain management clinic. Techniques such as cognitive behavioral therapy are an established means of helping people to manage long-term pain.

Unless a client has an acute and potentially dangerous neck condition, the general advice provided here is likely to be safe and helpful.

Recommendation	Rationale
Relative rest	Resting for more than 1 or 2 days is not usually helpful for people with neck pain.
Stay physically active	There are tremendous benefits for people with neck pain in staying physically active. Consider all forms of exercise that are deemed safe for that particular person, such as walking, swimming, and stretching classes. Remaining physically active does not have to involve formal exercise classes or sport. Walking to and from work or to and from the cinema, or to the shops instead of taking a car or public transport constitutes physical activity. Could your client do a home DVD exercise program? Could they walk their own dog or a friend's dog? Try to think "outside the box" and ask not what they cannot do, but what your client *can* do. How could you work with a fitness professional to help them increase their levels of physical activity? How could they increase this themselves on a daily basis?
Maintain active range of movement	While some people feel safer if they minimize the extent to which they move their head, in the long term, avoidance of all neck movements is not usually advisable as muscles atrophy with disuse and are therefore less able to support the head. Collars that keep the neck immobile are therefore not helpful in the long term. Even small movements can help reduce discomfort and improve recovery times.
Avoid aggravating factors	Help your client to identify which movements and activities most aggravate their neck. Consider ways to avoid or minimize these. For example, if they remain stationary for long periods of time, ask whether the task they are doing could be broken into smaller segments. Could they split up this activity throughout the day? Or, could they do some stretches or movements to overcome this static position.
Use heat or cold for pain relief	The application of heat and cold can be used for pain relief and which of them is used depends largely on the client's preferences. In acute situations, cold is usually applied, and it has a general numbing effect on the body and thus decreases pain. However, applying cold to the neck region is not always pleasant and could give some clients a headache. For this reason, it should be applied for a short duration only, for a few minutes if tolerable. Caution is needed to avoid using heat at too high a temperature or for too long a period. Heat is useful for decreasing muscle spasm, one of the contributing factors to pain. Performing neck ranges of movement or gentle neck stretches may be easier after the application of heat.

Recommendation	Rationale
Avoid feeling cold	When we are cold, we tend to shrug our shoulders and this increases the tone in neck muscles. It is therefore important to keep well wrapped up in cold weather and to identify risks such as when the client is in an air-conditioned environment. Some clients with neck pain are particularly susceptible to cold. What preventive measures do they take? Do they avoid certain environments? Carry a scarf? Carry a heat pack?
Encourage relaxation	Feeling stressed or angry increases muscle tone and is likely to aggravate some neck conditions. Finding ways to relax physically and emotionally is important in helping to manage neck conditions and helps aid recovery. Consider asking your client to think constructively about how they could build rest and relaxation into their rehabilitation program, just as they might plan neck exercises.

Tip 3: Get Clients Moving

The message here is that unless a client has suffered an acute injury, or has neck pain resulting from a serious pathology such as a herniated cervical disk, cervical fracture, or tumor, for example, movement and exercise is better for them than immobility.

| The Advantages of Activity and Disadvantages of Inactivity for People with Neck Pain ||
Advantages of activity	Disadvantages of inactivity
Helps maintain and improve range of movement in the neck	Is likely to lead to a decreased range of movement in the neck
May help reduce feelings of stiffness	Is likely to increase feelings of stiffness
May help reduce pain	May increase pain
Helps elevate a person's mood	May contribute to feelings of depression
Helps maintain and improve muscle strength	Results in muscles weakening
Helps maintain and improve proprioception in the joints of cervical vertebrae and can help maintain and improve balance	Is likely to lead to a reduction in proprioception in joints of cervical vertebrae and a reduction in balance
Movement promotes blood flow to muscles, tendons, and ligaments, aids lymph drainage and stimulates repair	Decreased blood flow to muscles, tendons, and ligaments combined with reduced lymph drainage is likely to increase scar tissue and hinder repair
Can help a client feel that they are in control and making progress	Can lead to feelings of helplessness and lack of progress

Advice for clients on how to incorporate neck movement into their daily activities without aggravating an existing neck condition	
Sleeping	On waking, lie on your back and gently roll your head from one side to the other. Next, sit on the edge of the bed and take your neck through its range of movement—flexion, extension, rotation left and right, and lateral flexion left and right, performing each movement one or two times. Neck and shoulder muscles are connected, so perform one or two shoulder shrugs or shoulder rolls. Together these movements can help get the joints of your neck moving and help you feel a little looser before you start your day.
Driving	Holding your head, neck, and shoulders stationary for long periods of time increases muscle tension and can aggravate certain neck conditions. Consider how to drive less—consider fewer journeys or journeys of shorter duration. Can you use other forms of transport or get a lift for all or some of your journey? If you have to drive, or have a particularly long journey planned, break up the journey as much as possible, stopping to rest. During these rests, perform simple range of movements such as neck movements, stretches, and shoulder shrugs or shoulder rolls. Adjust your seat so that you are as comfortable as possible before your journey.
Commuting and traveling	It is important to keep your neck moving, avoiding a static posture for long periods of time. Range of movement exercises and shoulder shrugs can be performed surreptitiously if you are concerned about people watching you, on a station platform or while waiting at an airport. If you need to travel on a crowded bus, train, or tram, sit if a seat is available so that you can avoid holding a bar or strap for support as elevation of the shoulder requires some neck and shoulder muscles to contract and shorten, and in some cases, this can lead to spasming of the muscle. This may be more likely to happen if you are prone to neck spasms. If you have to hold onto something by raising your arm, avoid using the arm on the side of your neck that spasms, or change arms where possible; practice depressing your shoulder blades a couple of times while you are holding on, contracting muscles opposite to those that are prone to spasm.

Advice for clients on how to incorporate neck movement into their daily activities without aggravating an existing neck condition	
Watching TV	Avoid remaining stationary without moving your neck for periods of more than about 40 min. Use commercial breaks as a prompt to perform simple neck movements and shoulder shrugs. Avoid sitting for long periods with your head turned to one side, even slightly. Is your TV screen in front of you or do you need to turn to watch it? Having to look up, to a wall-mounted screen, or down, to a screen close to the floor, for long periods of time increases muscle tension and is likely to aggravate certain neck conditions. Where possible, have your furniture rearranged so that your TV screen is in front of you and the top of the screen is level with your eyes.
Working at a desk	As with watching TV, avoid remaining stationary without moving your neck for periods of more than about 40 minutes. Do not wait to feel stiff and sore before moving. Move before that happens! Take regular micro breaks—30 seconds or so—and use these to perform simple neck movements and shoulder shrugs. Use a visual or auditory screen alert as a reminder for when it is time to take a break. Check that any screen you are using is in front of you and that the top of the screen is level with your eyes. Where possible, vary the type of work you are doing so that you change the position of your neck. For example, swap between typing and writing and speaking on the telephone. If you know that your neck starts to ache or spasm when in the draft from air conditioning or a window, get into the habit of always carrying a lightweight scarf with you that you can use as and when needed. Shoulder and neck muscles are connected, and overreaching for things on your desk could aggravate your neck condition. Move things closer to you where possible.
Hobbies	If a hobby requires you to keep your neck stationary for long periods of time, such as reading, needlework, painting, or fine model making, stop and take breaks every 40 minutes or so. Set a watch or phone alert to remind you when it is time to take a break during which you can move your neck and shoulders. Dog walkers report that sometimes a sharp tug on the leash can trigger their neck pain. Solutions are to swap the hand in which you hold the leash or to use an extendable leash.
Daily activities and chores	Lifting and carrying can aggravate some neck conditions as the load is transmitted through the arms and the shoulders to muscles spanning both the shoulder and the neck. Minimize what you need to lift and carry, carry items close to your body or not at all—use a wheelie case or buggy or backpack. When we carry a heavy bag on one shoulder, we tend to shrug that shoulder; this can aggravate some neck conditions and lead to spasming of the muscles on that side. If you have to carry a bag, try changing hands and swap the shoulder on which you carry it. Avoid holding a phone on one side of the head for long periods of time as such use tends to cause us to laterally flex to that side; this too can lead to spasming of muscles on that side. Where possible, minimize using the phone in this way or change the way you use it—convert to speakerphone, headset, or Skype, for example. Certain daily activities can trigger spasm in neck muscles where the activity involves lifting a weight on one side or raising one or both arms above the head, for example, holding a hair dryer to the head, reaching up to put crockery into a cupboard, reaching up to hang drapes, hanging washing on a line, reaching up to wash a window. In the acute stages, avoid these activities. Avoid or minimize time spent vacuuming or ironing, activities that involve repetitive movement of the arms combined with a fairly static neck posture.
Exercise and sports	Exercise and sports help people cope with pain, and help in the rehabilitation process. Impact and contact activities are potentially aggravating for people with neck conditions, so nonimpact and noncontact activities are preferable. Sports and exercise do not have to be stopped; they simply have to be modified. Ways to modify these are to change the activity itself (e.g., from cycling to walking), the intensity of the activity (e.g., every other day rather than every day), or the duration of the activity (e.g., 20 minutes a day instead of 60 minutes a day). Some activities can be modified to reduce their impact; for example, instead of doing breaststroke when swimming, change to backstroke.

Tip 4: **Simple Neck Stretches**

The most simple stretches you can give a client are active ROM stretches. Whilst ROM tests are used as part of cervical assessment, actively moving the neck through its normal ranges will constitute a stretch for some clients and they should practice these before attempting other stretches.

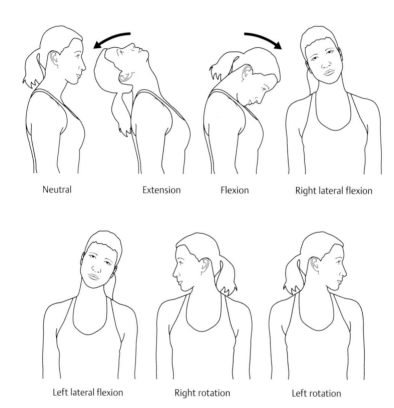

Neutral   Extension   Flexion   Right lateral flexion

Left lateral flexion   Right rotation   Left rotation

Follow this simple plan for increasing ROM in the neck:

1. Encourage your client to perform the movements of flexion, extension, right rotation, left rotation, right lateral flexion, and left lateral flexion, moving slowly, only as far into each range as they feel comfortable. Once the client is comfortable moving their neck, ask them to hold each position when they get to that point where they are starting to feel slight discomfort. Encourage them to repeat these movements throughout the day, following the maxim *little and often*.

2. Once the client is confident in attempting the ROMs movements, no matter how slight or how reduced in range, encourage them to increase the range slightly. Do this by suggesting that with each movement, as they approach the point at which they feel discomfort, they move gently 1 or 2 mm further into the range. This may be uncomfortable but should not hurt and if a client reports pain or dizziness, then of course they should stop.

Ask your client to practice these ROM stretches regularly throughout the day, and over the coming week to take note of any improvements. Improvements might come in the form of the following:

- Being able to move through a greater range.

- Being able to move through the same range with less pain.
- Being able to move through the same range with less hesitancy.
- Being able to move through the same range with less stiffness or less dizziness, etc.

Remember that it is important for the client to keep their shoulders still, not to twist at the waist or raise their shoulders to facilitate the movement.

It can be helpful to give a client a diary (example shown below) to complete which can act as a reminder and onto which they can note the following:

- Any increases in range.
- Any problems.
- How many times they were able to perform a particular movement.

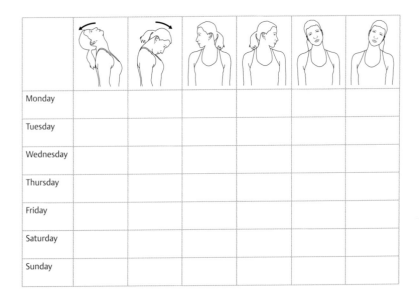

Monday						
Tuesday						
Wednesday						
Thursday						
Friday						
Saturday						
Sunday						

Alternative Ways to Increase Cervical Range of Movement

One way to increase active cervical rotation is for a client to lie on their back and to gently rotate their head to the left and to the right while it is supported by a bed or the floor.

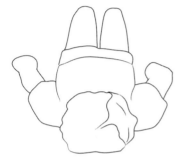

Another is for the client to apply gentle overpressure.

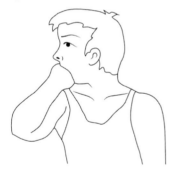

A third alternative is for a client to place a towel behind their head and, holding the ends of the towel, to use it to facilitate rotation themselves in either supine or sitting position.

Mulligan (2010) says that by hooking the selvage of the towel beneath the spinous process of a specific vertebra and applying gentle force upward and to one direction (e.g., right rotation or left rotation), the client can help mobilize that particular spinal segment. What do you think?

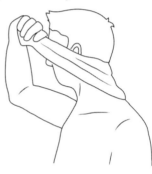

Tip 5: Enhancing Neck Stretches

Many therapists are used to providing simple stretches as part of their homecare advice to clients. It is worth considering whether you could enhance the stretch by making minor alterations to the stretch position. In the case of lateral flexion, altering the position of the shoulder or the head, or both, affects the part of the neck the stretch is felt and, depending on the tension in those tissues, the intensity of the stretch.

TIP: One of the things to consider when teaching clients how to stretch their necks is that as they lengthen the muscles on one side of their necks they shorten muscles on the opposite side. This means that the shortened muscles sometimes cramp. Cramp is easily overcome by simply stetching out that side of the neck. However, if you know a client is prone to right-sided torticollis, for example, they should avoid stretching the left lateral flexors as doing so could trigger spasming of the muscles on the right side of their neck.

Here are some examples of how you could alter a simple lateral neck stretch to more specifically target the tense tissues:

- Start with a simple lateral stretch in a neutral position. Take the head gently to the opposite side.

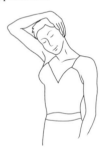

- Retaining this position, actively depress the shoulder by pressing the elbow toward the floor.

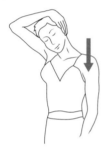

- Depress the shoulder by holding a chair prior to taking the head and neck into lateral flexion.

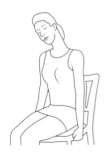

- Hold a light weight (such as a bag of shopping) prior to taking the head and the neck into lateral flexion.

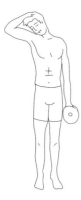

- Resting in the supine position, depress the shoulder and fix the arm beneath the body prior to taking the neck into lateral flexion.

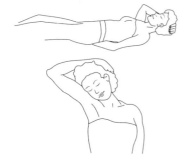

- Alter the arm position: abduct the shoulder.

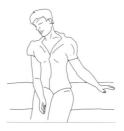

- Alter the arm: adduct the shoulder.

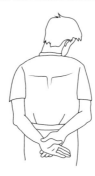

- Alter the head position and notice how you can focus the stretch more to the trapezius or to the levator scapulae. What position do you need to be in to move your head to get a better stretch of scalenes?

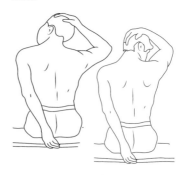

Tip 6: Neck Alignment while Sleeping

In Chapter 1, Tip 9 (p. 25), you learned how you could draw around a client in order to get a better understanding of the distance between their head and shoulders.

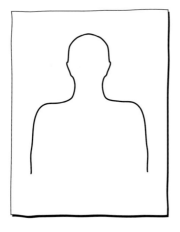

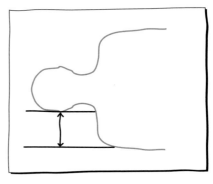

By turning the image above on its side, through 90 degrees, you can use it to help explain to a client what happens to their neck when they rest on their side with too many (or too fat) pillows (a) and too few (or too thin) pillows (b). You can use this image to demonstrate how, when a person has a neck condition, such positions can aggravate the symptoms by passively shortening the soft tissue on one side of the neck, in which case tissues on that side of the neck may cramp, while simultaneously lengthening the soft tissues on the other side of the neck, possibly overstretching them. Resting with the neck in lateral flexion in such a manner is not advisable. Using this same image from Chapter 1, Tip 9, you can demonstrate to the client that correctly filling the gap between their shoulder and head (c) can help keep the cervical spine in a more neutral alignment, a position where tissues are neither shortened nor lengthened and cervical vertebrae can remain unstressed.

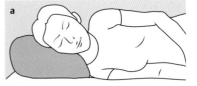

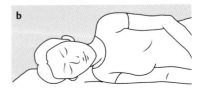

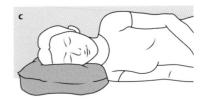

Tip 7: Neck Retractions

The center of gravity in humans falls slightly anterior to the transverse axis for flexion and extension of the head and neck. This means that our posterior neck muscles are active even when we are sitting or standing still, to prevent the head from falling forward. If you have ever seen anyone fall asleep on a train journey, you might have noticed that their head tends to fall forward or to the side, as the posterior muscles relax and the weight of gravity pulls the head downward. They may jerk suddenly, as the cervical stretch reflex kicks in, when spindles in muscle fibers detect stretch and signal to the muscle group to contract.

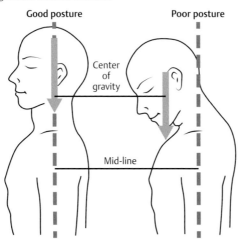

When we maintain a static posture that involves looking down slightly, as when writing, reading a book, or knitting, for example, our posterior neck muscles have to work hard to maintain our heads in this slightly flexed position, contracting eccentrically as we lower our heads into flexion, and concentrically to bring our heads back to the neutral position. They work even harder to bring about extension of the neck, as might be required when we look up to the ceiling when we are in the prone position. It is not suprising that many people experience tension and pain in their necks from the maintenance of static postures, and providing clients with an exercise they can do regularly to counteract this tension is highly beneficial. One such exercise is neck retraction.

This simple home care exercise is used to help clients with increased cervical lordosis and tension in the posterior neck muscles. It helps activate weakened deep neck flexors (longus colli and capitis). To perform neck retractions, a client needs to give themselves a double chin by pulling their head backward. They could look in the mirror to observe their neck or simply hold their hand on their chin as a guide.

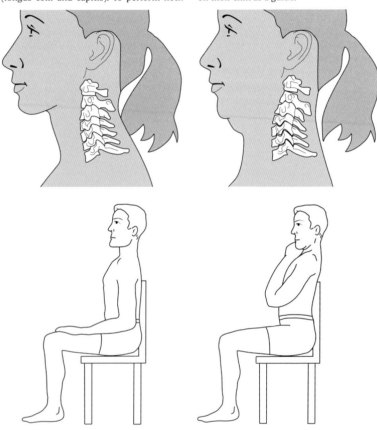

However, many clients find this difficult, so it is useful to practice first with them in supine on a treatment couch.

1. Place your finger in the midpoint of their neck, touching their skin.
2. Ask the client to try and push their neck back into your finger.
3. As you feel them doing this, slowly move your finger toward the treatment couch, thus making the client retract their head and neck a little more.

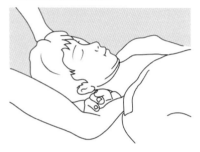

Use this exercise to explain the movement you need the client to perform while they are in a seated position.

In the seated position:

1. Suggest the client to imagine they have their chin resting on a shelf. This helps them keep their head facing forward. Without this command, some clients extend their head and neck—a movement you want to avoid.
2. Note that it is important for the client to avoid sustained maximal contraction of muscles as they bring about retraction. Ask them to "relax off" just a little so that they have changed the position of their head and neck, yet are avoiding maximal contraction of scalenes.

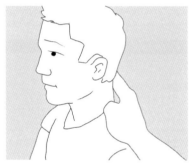

Tip 8: **Trigger Point Massage**

Using a spikey hard rubber or plastic therapy ball, clients can learn to treat trigger points all over their bodies, including the back of their necks where they can access the neck extensors.

Question: Are there any clients for whom self-triggering is contraindicated?

Clients with acute conditions, such as osteoporosis, rheumatoid arthritis, or another cervical condition that is contraindicated for massage, should avoid this treatment. Care should be taken by clients who bruise easily and all clients should be advised that they are aiming to reduce tension in the muscles of their necks, and so should avoid pressing hard onto the bones of their neck.

The following table contrasts the advantages and disadvantages of using a therapy ball to deactivate trigger points in two different treatment positions—standing and supine.

	Standing	Supine
Advantages	• This is a good starting point to experiment with how the client will respond to self-management of trigger points, as the client can choose how much pressure they exert against the ball. • This is useful for when the client wants to use the ball during the day, at work for example. • The ball can be gently rolled up and down using simple nodding movement of the head, to access the suboccipital muscles.	• The client can relax almost completely, letting their head roll side to side. • This means that as tissues relax they may be able to access deeper soft tissue structures with the pressure of the ball. • Some clients find it easier to access muscles to one side of their posterior neck in this way, as they can rest with their head in slight rotation.
Disadvantages	• It can be difficult to keep the ball in place. • It requires pressing through muscles which are actively engaged in order to keep the head erect and may therefore decrease the effectiveness of accessing deeper muscles such as suboccipitals. • Some clients may find their quadriceps fatigue from having to make constant squatting movements as they maneuver the ball into place. • It can be difficult to move the ball left to right. • If a client is particularly kyphotic or even just a little round-shouldered, it can be difficult getting close enough to the wall to access the back of the neck in this way.	• It can be difficult to access a trigger point above or below the point at which they are working as this means maneuvering themselves off the floor so that they can roll superior or inferior and onto the required trigger. • The head is heavy and for some people there is a danger that this is too much pressure and they risk overtreating, so good advice is to suggest that a client practice for a few minutes and see how their tissues respond the following day.

How to Use a Therapy Ball to Help Deactivate Trigger Points

The illustrations on the following page show sites of common trigger points. Triggers are tender to touch and develop over many months or even years. Retention of a static upper body posture is thought to contribute to the development of trigger points in muscles of the neck. To treat these using a ball, gently press the ball onto the trigger point for about 30 seconds. The sensation should be slightly uncomfortable but not painful. Importantly, with gentle pressure this sensation should subside. When it subsides, press gently again into the trigger point. Further discomfort should subside within about 60 seconds. Repeat about three times. Rub or massage the area following use of the ball. If the discomfort does not subside, do not apply further pressure. If, the following day, your neck feels sore or is bruised, you should not attempt trigger point work again. If, as is usually the case, your symptoms feel somewhat relieved, you can use the ball again, in the same manner.

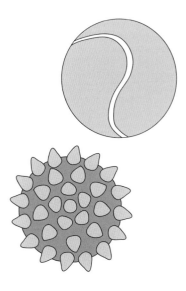

Examples of common trigger points in the neck

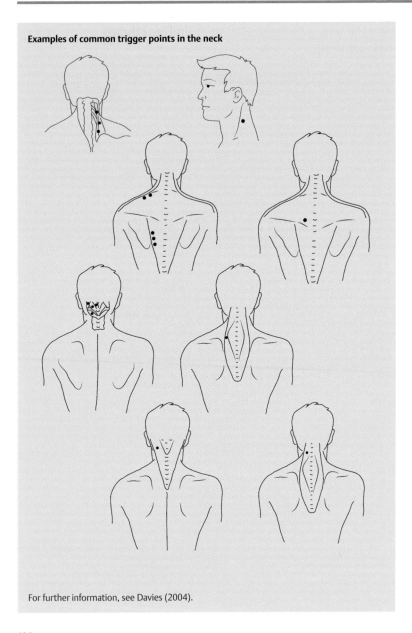

For further information, see Davies (2004).

Tip 9: A Trick with the Eyes!

This active technique improves cervical rotation. Practice on yourself first to see how it works.

To Increase Rotation to the Right

1. Turn your head to the **right** as far as you can.

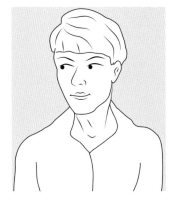

2. With your head in this position, move your eyes as far as you can to the **left**. Hold for 10 seconds.

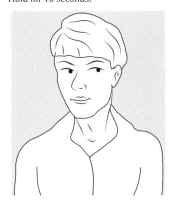

3. Now look **right** and notice that you gain a few millimeters in right cervical rotation.

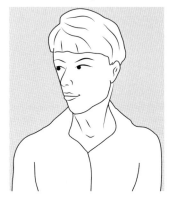

When teaching clients, remember to observe their cervical ROM both before and after this activity.

To Increase Rotation to the Left

1. Turn your head to the **left** as far as you can.

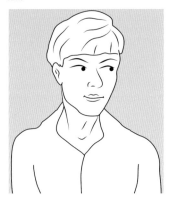

3. Now look **left** and notice that you gain a few millimeters in left cervical rotation.

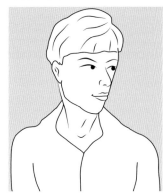

2. With your head in this position, move your eyes as far as you can to the **right**. Hold for 10 seconds.

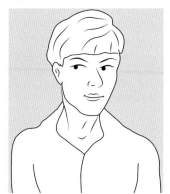

Tip 10: **Self-Massage**

Using the examples shown here, teaching your client how to self-massage their neck can be very helpful.

a Squeezing the occipital region

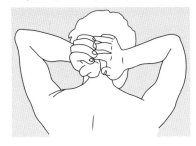

b Stroking or gripping neck extensors

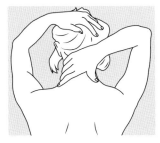

c Using a theracane for trigger point work

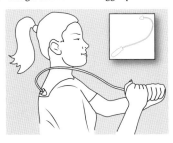

d Using a broom handle for upper trapezius

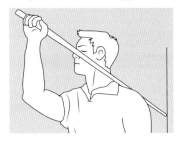

e Gentle massage to scalenes

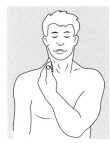

f Using thumbs to massage suboccipitals

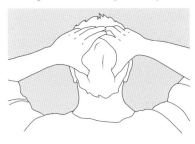

Tip 11: **Strengthening the Neck**

Isometric strengthening exercises are used for strengthening weak muscles. Shown here are some of the simplest exercises. Isometric strengthening can be done in these positions using bands, pulleys, and weights but are not shown here. Such advanced isometric exercises could cause harm if performed without supervision.

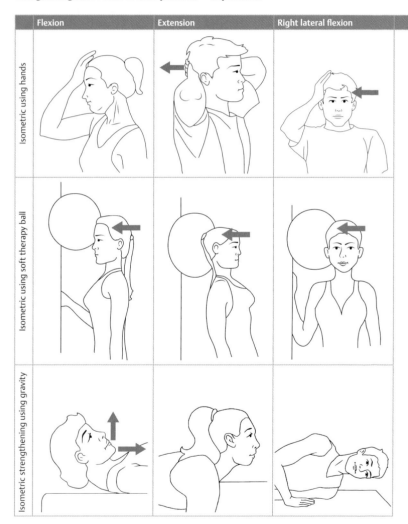

	Flexion	Extension	Right lateral flexion
Isometric using hands			
Isometric using soft therapy ball			
Isometric strengthening using gravity			

	Left lateral flexion	Right rotation	Left rotation
Isometric using hands			
Isometric using soft therapy ball			
Isometric strengthening using gravity			

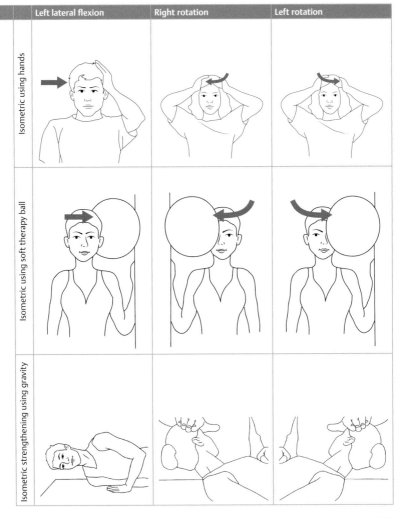

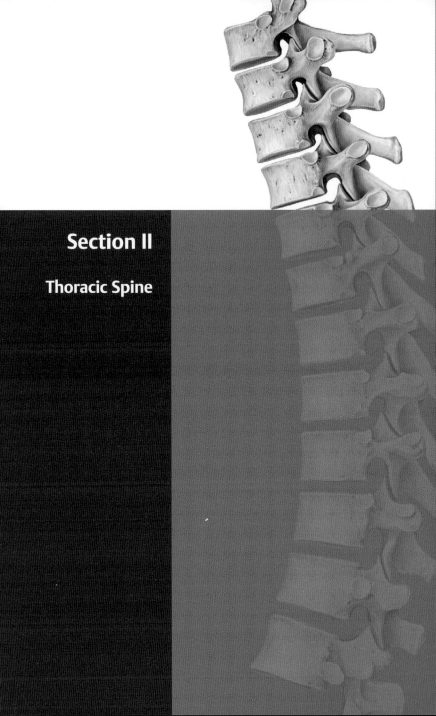

Section II

Thoracic Spine

Introduction

Many people suffer from thoracic back pain. Chronic pain is common in people who maintain prolonged, static postures whilst acute pain often accompanies injury. The challenge facing us as therapists is lack of evidence regarding best assessment and treatment approaches. The aim of this section of the book is to share tests and treatments you may find useful in your practice. You may feel inspired to select one tip and practice using it for many months, as and when you feel it appropriate, or you may wish to discuss several tips with a colleague or fellow student: what are the practicalities of the tip, its pros and cons? You may dislike some of the tips provided here and find them cumbersome; other tips may be known to you already. However, it is hoped that there is more than one tip that will inspire your curiosity and fire your enthusiasm. By sharing and collating information, we can all contribute to the (relatively) limited body of knowledge concerning this important part of the spine.

The tips provided here are effective and safe. They fall within the remit of qualified therapists. If you are a newly qualified therapist or have not practiced for some time, the information you find here will improve your understanding and help you to gain confidence.

It is assumed that you have consulted your client and taken their general medical history, that you have decided that your client is safe to be assessed and treated, and that they have given consent for this.

Each of the three chapters in this section is made up of numbered tips. You will also discover, embedded in the text, additional tips. Common questions and answers are included in boxes.

Chapter IV

Thoracic Assessment

Chapter 4 **Thoracic Assessment**

Many of you would have come across clients with pain in the upper part of their back, the thoracic spine. This is sometimes present in the thorax alone, but is often accompanied by symptoms in the neck or lumbar spine. Symptoms range from feelings of stiffness to burning muscular pain, pain often associated with the retention of static postures. Assessment of the region which links the cervical and lumbar spines is crucial and yet overlooked by many therapists.

Twenty six assessment tips provided here include simple identification of bony landmarks, palpation, and range of movement (ROM) tests that you may be familiar with, but also includes unique ways to test for thoracic stiffness, rib excursion, and some quick tests to help you assess muscle length. A systematic approach to assessment is encouraged, but you do not need to use all of these assessments with each client.

These are safe assessments for most people with thoracic symptoms. However, as a practicing therapist you will no doubt be able to determine for yourself their appropriateness. For example, Adam's test for scoliosis requires a subject to bend over, flexing at the waist. You would not wish someone with problems in their lumbar spine to do this, nor someone who experiences dizziness in such a position. Similarly, you would not wish to "rock" individual vertebrae to assess their mobility in a subject with osteoporosis or rheumatoid arthritis. These are commonsense contraindications, about which you are likely to be aware of. Nevertheless, where special caution is needed, this is noted in the text.

Tip 1: Identifying Key Bony Landmarks

Some of the methods of assessment described in the tips in this chapter require you to locate specific bones. For example, in Tip 2, it will be useful to be able to identify the T12/L1 junction as well as the iliac crest; in Tip 3, you will need to identify the medial border and the inferior angle of the scapula; in Tip 15, you will have to locate the 10th thoracic vertebra (T10). Many other tips refer to bony landmarks. Identifying these bones on an illustration is easier than locating them on a live subject. So let us begin with some tips to help you quickly locate these landmarks.

The thoracic column is joined to the neck at C7/T1, where the first thoracic vertebra (T1) joins the seventh thoracic vertebra (C7). The junction of the thoracic column and the lumbar spine is at T12/L1, where the 12th thoracic vertebra (T12) joins the first lumbar vertebra (L1).

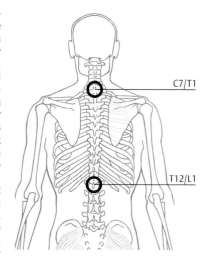

Locating C7

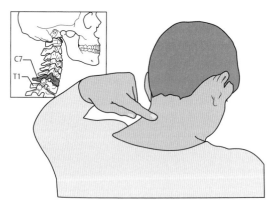

C7 is the most prominent vertebra of the cervical spine. In standing or sitting positions, it can be located simply by flexing the head and the neck: the most prominent "bump" on the back of the neck is the spinous process of this vertebra. In some people, this bump is very obvious; in others, it is less so. C7 moves on movement of the neck.

Locating T1: The First Thoracic Vertebra

Once you have identified C7, simply palpate inferior to this point to try to locate the spinous process of the first thoracic vertebra, T1, the beginning of the thoracic spine.

Although you may feel some soft tissue changes, T1 itself moves less than C7 with movement of the neck.

TIP: Place your hand on the back of your neck and see if you can identify C7 and T1 by moving your neck and identify which of the vertebrae move the most. Try this on a colleague.

Locating T12: The 12th Thoracic Vertebra

Instead of having to "count down" every single spinous process from the occiput until you reach the 12th thoracic vertebra, remember that T12 has a floating rib attached to it on each side. Therefore, if you locate the 12th rib, it will be relatively easy to locate T12. Be careful as you palpate here, for, as you know, the kidneys lie in this region. The 12th rib can be difficult to find, but the 11th rib is more easily palpated and rests approximately horizontal with the spinous process of T12.

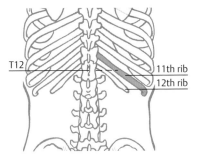

There are three positions in which you can do this.

The first position is with your subject standing. Ask him or her to abduct their arms a little and place your hands against the back of their rib cage. Palpate until you think you have found the lowest ribs. Then bring your hands inward, trying to differentiate between soft tissue and bone. The disadvantage of this method is that you are palpating through the thoracolumbar fascia and active erector spinae muscles. Also, when standing, your subject will have a tendency to lean back toward you in order to maintain balance as you palpate and this will further increase the tone in their muscles. You will also need to kneel or sit behind your subject to avoid stooping.

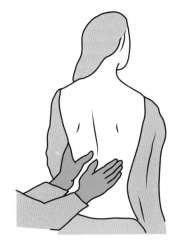

The second position is with your client straddling a chair, perhaps with a pillow between their stomach and the chair back. This helps your subject relax and decreases tone in the spinal extensor muscles slightly, but again you will need to sit or kneel behind your subject.

The third position is with your client prone. With your client in this position, the tone in the muscles of spinal extension is decreased and it is easier to palpate through them, to the ribs. Notice that the ribs are angled downward, so you will need to guestimate T12 as being slightly superior to the position in which you locate the lowest ribs.

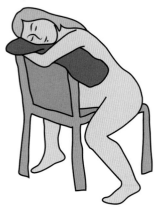

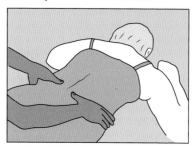

Locating the Iliac Crest

With your subject either standing or prone, gently squeeze their waist with the web of your hand. Press your hands downward and when you hit bony resistance on either side, that is the iliac crest.

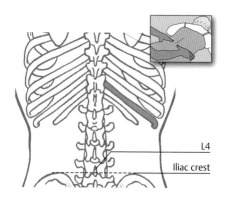

L4

Iliac crest

Locating L4

With your hands on the iliac crest, extend your thumbs and try to get your thumb tips to touch. Your thumb tips are pointing toward L4. Some people have an extra lumbar vertebra, in which case this assessment will be inaccurate, but for the general population this is a crude but useful way to locate L4. Once you have located L4, you can palpate superiorly to the spinous process of L3, L2, and L1, or inferiorly to L5.

Locating the Medial Border and Inferior Angle of the Scapula

On many people the scapula is prominent and its outline readily visible. On others, it may be difficult to distinguish due to overlying musculature or an excess of body fat. One quick way to identify the scapula is simply to ask your subject to place their hand behind their back. In doing so, the medial border and inferior angle of this bone become more prominent. Remember, however, as soon as your subject lowers their arm, the scapula position will change and become less prominent again. So use the test to identify the scapula but not to record its resting position.

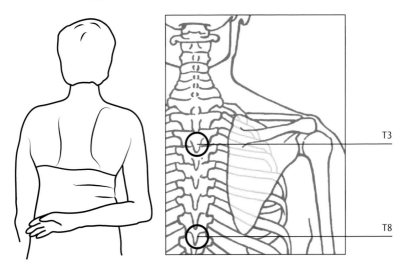

The inferior angle rests approximately level with the spinous process of T8, the spine of the scapula approximately level with T3, and it has been suggested that the medial borders should be approximately 5 cm (2 in) lateral to the spinous processes of the spine.

Locating a Transverse Process

Look at this cross section of the back of the thorax.

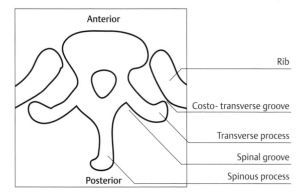

The spinous process is the most central bony protrusion. Place your finger or thumb on your subject's spinous process. Now glide gently to one side of this and you will feel a dip. This is the spinal groove formed by the transverse process of that vertebra. If you slide your finger or thumb ever so slightly more laterally, you will feel the protrusion of the tip of the transverse process.

Locating Rib Articulations

If you glide even more laterally, you can feel the costotransverse groove, a useful point to be able to locate when trying to determine whether ribs are correctly aligned.

TIP: You are working through contracted muscles if you palpate while your subject is seated or standing, and through relaxed muscles if you palpate with your subject prone.

Locating Rib Angles

Rib angles are the most prominent parts of the ribs. They can be felt with the palm of your hand and seen when a person crosses their arms and flexes slightly at the waist. There is more information about this in Tip 22: Assessing Ribs (pp. 209–210).

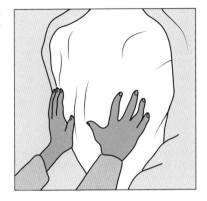

Tip 2: Thoracolumbar Junction Syndrome (Maigne Syndrome)

Although this section is about the thorax, as a therapist you know that body parts cannot be easily compartmentalized and that they impact on one another. This tip has been included near the start of the assessment section because it helps reinforce this point. In 1974, Robert Maigne studied the phenomenon of pain referred from the T10–T11, T11–T12, and T12–L1 regions of the spine.

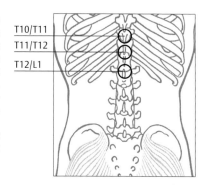

Maigne (1974) noted that nerves exiting the T12/L1 segment of the spine can refer pain to the following:

- The posterior iliac crest.
- The greater trochanter.
- The groin.

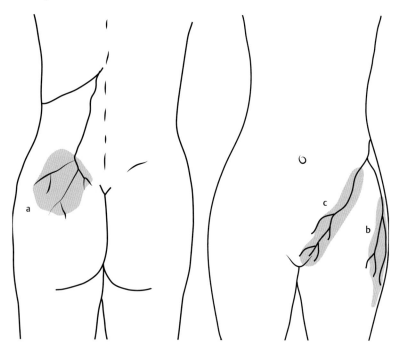

He speculated that problems may arise in this particular segment of the spine because it is where a vertebra with the ability to rotate (the last thoracic vertebra, T12) joins a vertebra with almost no rotation (the first lumbar vertebra, L1).

How did Maigne suggest we identify a client with symptoms in their buttock, greater trochanter, or groin as suffering from thoracolumbar joint syndrome?

First, Maigne observed that if you apply gentle lateral pressure to the spinous processes (a), T12 to L2 will be uncomfortable when pressure is applied to the affected segment.

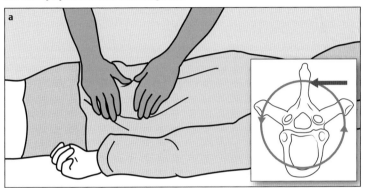

Second, he said cellulalgia will be present. Cellulalgia describes an area of thickened skin where skin rolling (b) elicits tenderness. The area in which these symptoms occur corresponds to the spinal nerve involved. If the thoracolumbar junction is involved, you would expect a thickening of skin in the iliac crest/superior buttock region.

Third, you would be able to reproduce symptoms when a point that is 7–8 cm (2.7–3.1 in) from the midline on the iliac crest (c) is rubbed, as this is where the associated cutaneous T11, T12, or L1 nerve crosses the ilium. For two interesting case studies, see Proctor et al (1985).

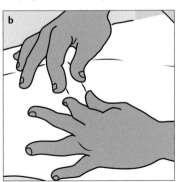

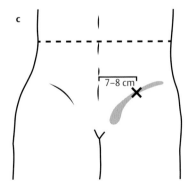

Tip 3: Postural Assessment of the Thoracic Region – A Reminder

On the next few pages are some questions that serve as a reminder of some of the key aspects to consider when carrying out a postural assessment of the thoracic region. Postural assessment of the upper body includes an assessment of the head and neck, so remember to observe your client's head position, especially whether they have a forward head posture, as this affects how thoracic muscles function. You will need to examine all aspects of your subject's thorax, observing them from the front, back, and side.

Question: Does it matter where I start my assessment—anterior, lateral, or posterior?

No. However, some clients might feel anxious if you were to start by facing them. Many people have never had their posture assessed and for a client to stand, semi-clothed, for an anterior postural assessment could feel intimidating.

Posterior View

Is the rib cage centered over the pelvis or is there evidence of thoracic rotation, lateral flexion, or lateral shift (a)?

Does the spine appear fairly straight or is there any evidence of scoliosis (b)? For how to assess for scoliosis, please see Tip 6 (pp. 163–166).

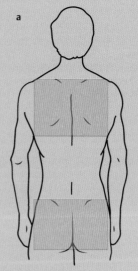

a

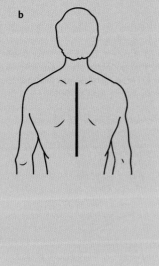

b

Are the scapulae equidistant from the spine or is there evidence of abduction (protraction) (c) or adduction (retraction) (d)?

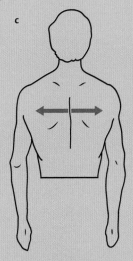

TIP: You could measure the distance of the medial border from the spine.

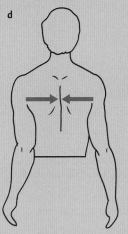

Are the shoulders level or does one appear raised and one dropped? Examine the inferior angle to assess for elevation (e) or depression (f) of either scapula.

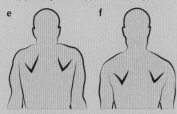

If there is asymmetry, is this due to the position of the shoulder itself or to an increase/decrease in bulk in elevators of the shoulder such as the upper fibers of trapezius (not shown)?

Is there any evidence of either upward or downward rotation of the scapulae (g)?

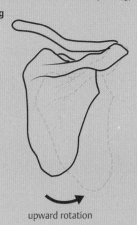

upward rotation

Is there evidence of scapular winging (h)? For more information, see Tip 5 (p. 162). How do the ribs appear? Are they symmetrical (i)? Do any rib angles appear particularly prominent?

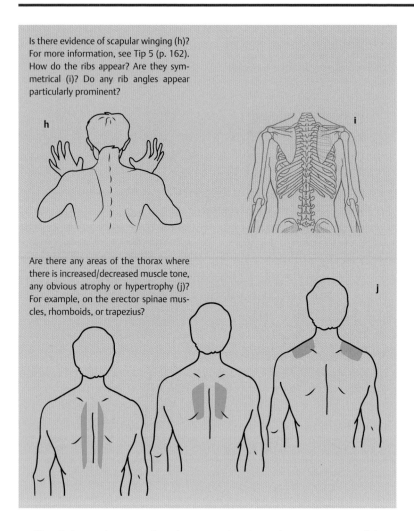

Are there any areas of the thorax where there is increased/decreased muscle tone, any obvious atrophy or hypertrophy (j)? For example, on the erector spinae muscles, rhomboids, or trapezius?

Although their study was specific to the assessment of musicians, Struyf et al (2009) provide a nice overview of the assessment of scapula position.

Lateral View

Is there evidence of a forward head posture (a)?

How does the cervicothoracic junction appear—any sign of a dowager's hump (b)?

Is there evidence of kyphosis or flat back (c)? For more information on flat back, see Tip 4.

Is the thorax elevated or depressed? Is the person slouched or standing with a military posture (d)?

Any evidence of scapular tipping (e)?

Are the shoulders abducted (protracted) or adducted (retracted)?

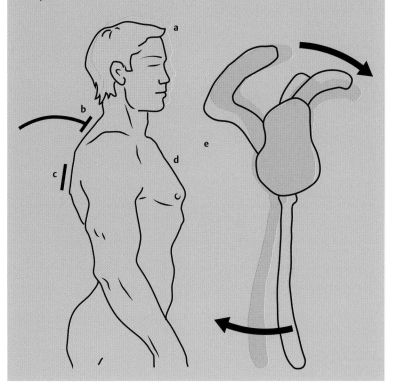

Anterior View

Is the thorax centralized over the pelvis (a)?

How does the muscle tone on pectorals (b) and abdomen (c) appear?

What is the position of the clavicles (d)? Clavicles indicate the position of the scapulae which attach to these bones at the acromioclavicular joint. Is there evidence of shoulder elevation or depression or protraction or retraction based on your observation of the clavicles?

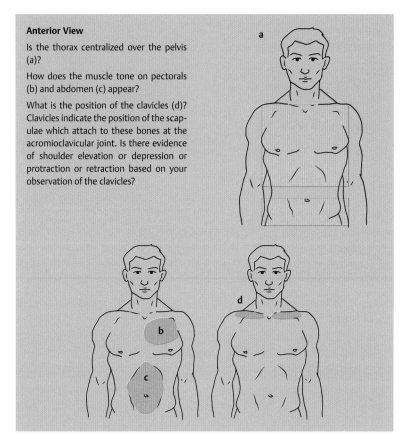

For a full description of how to perform postural assessment, including what your findings might mean, please see Johnson (2012).

Tip 4: Assessing for Flat Back

One of the key things to observe in a thoracic assessment is whether or not your subject has the normal thoracic curve. Many therapists are quick to spot kyphotic postures, and it is equally important to assess for a flat back. A flattened thoracic curve can contribute to localized pain. Observe how the spinous process of a normal thoracic vertebra points downward. Loss of the thoracic curve means that these processes come closer together. Sometimes, clients with flat back complain of pain on standing erect, and even greater pain on extension of their spine. Of course, it is important to rule out other causes of this pain, but pain could be the result of the soft tissues and spinous processes being jammed together on movements involving spinal extension.

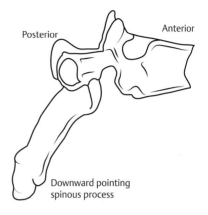

Posterior

Anterior

Downward pointing
spinous process

Tip 5: **Scapular Winging**

True scapular winging is observed as a marked protrusion of the scapula from the posterior chest wall. It is unlike the mild protrusion of scapulae you sometimes see in a client with low body fat, or the slightly more prominent appearance of the scapulae in a client with a flat back. True scapular winging is the result of nerve palsy, frequently affecting the serratus anterior muscle so that it cannot hold the scapula against the rib cage. This may be due to a congenital abnormality or may be the result of injury to the long thoracic nerve.

Weakness in trapezius and rhomboids can also contribute to scapular instability. Shortening of pectoralis minor could tilt the scapula anteriorly, making the inferior angle more prominent.

For a good overview, see Martin and Fish (2008).

For a brief and interesting overview of patients treated surgically for scapular winging, see Iceton and Harris (1987).

Question: How can I tell if my client has true scapular winging?

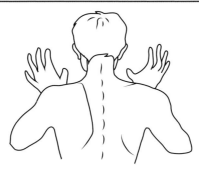

Ask your client to rest their hands against a wall and attempt to extend their elbows as if doing a push-up against the wall. Serratus anterior functions to bring about protraction and also to stabilize the scapulae against the chest wall during this push-up action. If the scapulae "wing" away from the chest wall during the activity, this indicates serratus anterior is weak or nonfunctioning. If it is nonfunctioning, then the scapulae will wing even if the subject is standing, without having to perform a push-up.

Tip 6: **Adam's Test for Scoliosis**

The S-shaped lateral curvature of the spine known as scoliosis is varied and requires a specialist to diagnose the type and degree of the problem. Many people have spines with mild deviation from the midline, but these would not be described as scoliotic.

There are two types of scoliosis: functional and structural.

In *functional scoliosis*, sometimes called flexible scoliosis, there are no structural changes to vertebrae or pathology affecting ligaments or muscles.

Structural scoliosis, sometimes called rigid scoliosis, involves changes to the vertebrae.

William Adams (1820–1900) devised the forward bending test, which carries his name.

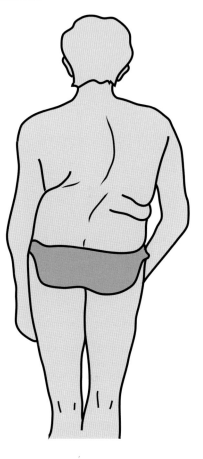

Using the Adam's Test

Ask your subject to bend forward as far as they are able as you observe their rib cage.

A rib "hump" is revealed on the side of their spine that is convex.

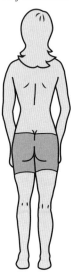
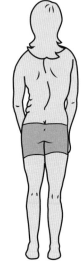
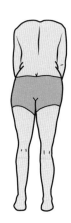
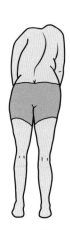

In very general terms, *functional* scoliosis disappears on the Adam's test (forward flexion) and on lying supine, and may be corrected by the subject. *Structural* scoliosis does not disappear on the Adam's test—if anything, this test highlights the scoliosis; the scoliosis does not disappear when the subject rests supine and the curve cannot be corrected by the subject without assistance.

Generalized overview comparing functional and structural scoliosis

	Functional scoliosis	Structural scoliosis
Adam's test	Disappears	Remains or is more prominent
Resting supine	Disappears	Resting supine is often possible but may be uncomfortable as scoliosis remains
Can be corrected independently by the subject	YES	NO

In the scoliotic spine, as the body of a thoracic vertebra starts to rotate counterclockwise (as it would with lateral flexion to the right), its spinous process moves counterclockwise also, appearing to the right of the midline. The ribs, attached to the vertebrae, also move: they become convex on the anterior, right side of the body, and convex on the posterior, left side of the body.

Normal thorax (a) and thorax in scoliotic subject flexing to the right (b).

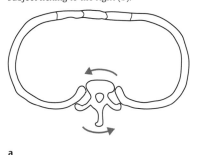
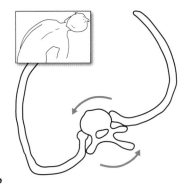

a   b

Changes in vertebrae and ribs associated with lateral flexion to the right or to the left, as you are standing behind the subject are shown in the following table.

	Lateral flexion to the right	Lateral flexion to the left
Movement of vertebral bodies	Counterclockwise to the left	Clockwise to the right
Movement of spinous processes	Counterclockwise to the right of the midline	Clockwise to the left of the midline
Posterior ribs	Project on the left of the body	Project on the right of the body
Anterior ribs	Project on the right of the body	Project on the left of the body
Thoracic cage	Thoracic cage reduced on left side of body	Thoracic cage reduced on right side of body

Question: How can I measure the degree of scoliosis in order to help determine if my interventions have been helpful?

There are many different ways to do this. Fairbank (2004) gives a nice account of a subject, Giddeon Mantell, whom Adams identified as having scoliosis. For a good article describing how to use more detailed measurements to assess scoliosis, please see Petias et al (2010). Alternatively, consider the simple exercise described on the following page.

Measuring the Degree of Scoliosis

A simple method for measuring the degree of scoliosis is to place markers on various bony landmarks, using photographs taken before and after your intervention, and examine the markers to determine to what extent your intervention has affected the scoliotic posture of your subject.

Examples of useful bony landmarks you could use include the following:

1. The spinous process of C7.
2. The spinous process of L4.
3. The superior angle of the scapula.
4. The inferior angle of the scapula.
5. The acromion (not shown).
6. The posterior superior iliac spines.

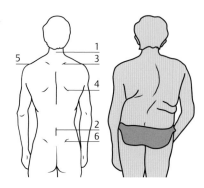

Note that this would only provide information about the change in relationship between body parts. You may wish to examine whether your intervention has had an impact on functional changes, such as improvements to respiratory capacity or a person's ability to perform daily activities, for example.

Question: Does it matter where you stand when carrying out the Adam's test assessment?

The Adam's test is usually performed with the observer standing behind their subject. However, this could make some subjects feel uncomfortable. If you stand in front of your client, you can still observe whether they have evidence of scoliosis.

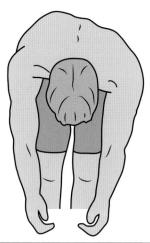

Tip 7: A Trick for Identifying Spine Shape

In complete contrast to the assessments for scoliosis in the previous tip, this trick is a crude and unorthodox method for quickly assessing the shape of the spine posteriorly. Gently run the side of your fingernail down each side of the subject's spine, leaving a faint track mark on the skin—but obviously not breaking the skin. Then stand back and observe the tracks you have made. Deviations from vertical are sometimes immediately apparent in this crude and quick assessment.

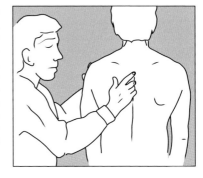

Tip 8: Assessing Thoracic Range of Movement

Being able to assess whether a client has a hypomobile or hypermobile thoracic spine is useful as increased or decreased mobility in this part of the spine can cause or contribute to pain. However, unlike the cervical region of the spine, it can be difficult to accurately assess range of movement (ROM) in the thorax. When testing cervical ROM, you may instruct your client to look left or right, up to the ceiling or down to the floor, or to take their ear toward their shoulder. Performing the corresponding movements of rotation, flexion, extension, and lateral flexion in the thoracic spine is difficult to achieve in isolation as these movements are accompanied by movements in the lumbar spine too:

- Lateral flexion of the thorax is accompanied by lumbar rotation to the opposite side.
- Thoracic rotation is accompanied by lumbar lateral flexion to the opposite side.

Thoracic and lumbar movements

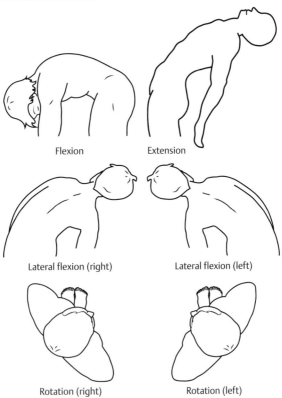

Flexion   Extension

Lateral flexion (right)   Lateral flexion (left)

Rotation (right)   Rotation (left)

There is disagreement as to the best method of assessing ROM in the thoracic (and lumbar) spine. The simplest way is to observe the movements your client can achieve. You might do this if you wanted to know which movement provoked a particular symptom rather than how much motion was available.

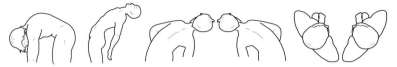

To assess ROM visually, demonstrate the six movements you wish your subject to perform and then observe as they perform the movements for themselves. Then, using the table showing normal ROMs (see p. 170), decide whether you think your subject has an increased or decreased ROM in their thoracic spine.

When assessing flexion, what do you think might impair ROM when your subject is tested in the standing position? Could it be tension in soft tissues of the hamstrings and calf? Or even the cervical and lumbar regions posteriorly? Might there be balance issues?

Question: Does it matter which movement the client performs first?

No. If you are new to using ROM tests, and when you are first practicing, it is always useful to ask clients to perform the movements in the same order. That way you are unlikely to miss out any movement. However, as you become more experienced, one tip is to leave the movement that you think might be most aggravating until last. You are likely to have some idea as to which movement this might be based on what your client has told you during your consultation. Note that you will need to stand to the side of your client in order to observe the movements of flexion and extension.

TIP: Hertling and Kessler (1996) say that subjects tend to fix their eyes on a spot on the floor and use their vision to guide forward flexion. They suggest that by asking a client to perform flexion with their eyes shut, any drift (to the right or to the left) will be more apparent. What do you think?

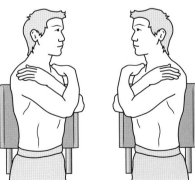

TIP: When assessing rotation, compare the results of your subject standing to sitting. In sitting, the pelvis is fixed so your results reflect more accurately the degree of rotation, which can appear greater when a subject is standing.

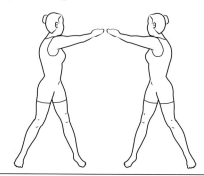

TIP: With all ROMs, watch for cheating movements, e.g., a subject who flexes slightly in order to achieve rotation.

TIP: Rotation requires deformation of the costal cartilages and as we age, these begin to ossify. This ossification is one of the factors contributing to reduced thoracic rotation in older adults.

The tips that follow provide you with ideas for measuring ROM in the thoracic spine, using a tape measure (Tip 9, pp. 171–177) and a goniometer (Tip 11, pp. 181–185). Consider them and decide which you feel might work best for you.

	Normal thoracic ROM[a]
Flexion	80–90 degrees
Extension	20–30 degrees
Lateral flexion	20–35 degrees
Rotation	30–45 degrees

Abbreviation: ROM, range of movement.
[a]Data from Greene and Heckman (1994).

Tip 9: Measuring Thoracic ROM Using a Tape Measure

One way to assess ROM in the thoracic spine is with skin distraction. This involves placing a tape measure against two standard points of reference and measuring by how much these points move apart or by how much they come closer together. The two points of reference you will need to identify are the spinous process of the 7th cervical vertebra (C7) and the spinous process of the 12th tho- racic vertebra (T12). Once you have located these positions you can position a tape mea- sure between them and measure the changes that occur as a subject flexes or extends.

Tip 12 (pp. 186–188) shows the measure- ment changes you might expect in a normal, healthy individual. Practice taking your own measurements first before consulting the table, so that your results are not prejudiced.

Measuring Thoracic Flexion: Method 1

Decide and document in which position your client will perform the movement: standing, sitting, or side lying.

STEP 1 Locate C7 and T12 on your subject.

STEP 2 Measure the distance between these two points and record your findings.

STEP 3 Ask the client to flex, and measure the distance between C7 and T12 again. Note the dif- ference between your first (neutral) and second (flexed) readings and record your findings again.

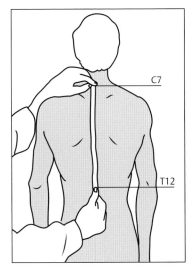

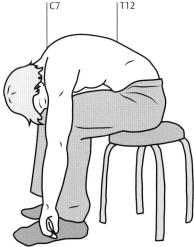

Question: Does it matter whether my subject is sitting or standing when I assess them?

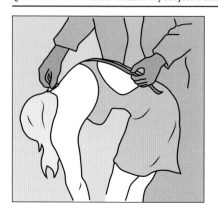 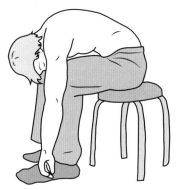

You are likely to get different results using different assessment positions. In *sitting*, the lumbar spine cannot fully flex, so if you were to measure the thorax only, a sitting position might be preferable. However, if a client is overweight or with large breasts or abdomen, they may find it uncomfortable to achieve full flexion while seated. While the lumbar spine is capable of fuller flexion in the *standing position* than in the sitting position, the muscles and fascia of the back of the body—especially the lower limbs—can restrict movement. Completing the tables under Tip 10 will help you identify the effect of different test positions on your results.

TIP: If you choose to measure flexion in standing, the pelvis should be stabilized to prevent anterior tilting. However, this makes measurement difficult unless there is one person to stabilize the subject's pelvis and another to use the tape measure.

Measuring Thoracic Flexion: Method 2

Another way to measure flexion is to measure the distance between the floor and the tip of your client's middle finger (a), or how far down their tibia they can reach (b). How reliable do you think this method is? What factors might influence your findings?

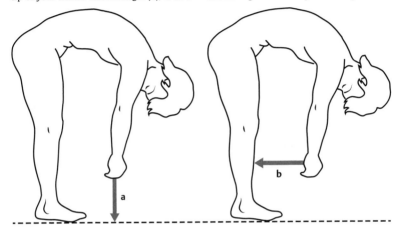

Measuring Thoracic Extension with a Tape Measure

Decide and document in which position your client will perform the movement: standing, sitting, or prone.

STEP 1 Locate C7 and T12 on your subject.

STEP 2 Measure the distance between these two points and record your findings.

STEP 3 Ask the client to extend, and measure the distance between C7 and T12 again. Note the difference between your first (neutral) and second (extended) readings and again record your findings.

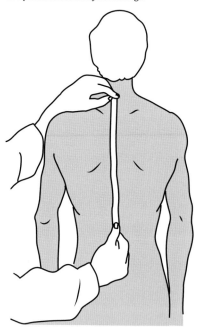
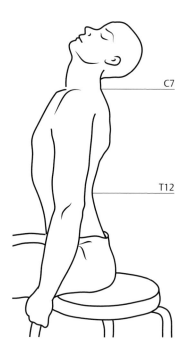

Measuring Lateral Flexion with a Tape Measure: Method 1

STEP 1 Ask your client to place their hands by their sides, their palms touching their thighs. Measure the distance between the tip of your client's middle finger and the floor, as they are standing erect.

STEP 2 Ask your client to bend to one side, performing lateral flexion. Measure the distance from your client's middle finger as it rests against their thigh to the floor.

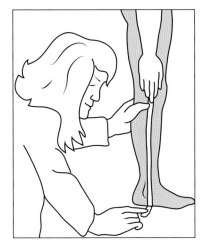

TIP: Other methods are to measure the distance from the start position to the head of the fibula, or to measure the distance of the fingertip from the knee joint each time. How accurate do you think these methods are? What factors might alter your results?

Measuring Lateral Flexion with a Tape Measure: Method 2

Moll and Wright (1981) suggest placing two marks on the lateral side of the thorax, one parallel with the xiphoid process of the sternum and the other at the most superior point of the iliac crest.

Then, when your subject laterally flexes, you can measure either by how far the distance is reduced on the side to which they flex (a) or by how far the marks are distracted on the opposite side of their body (b).

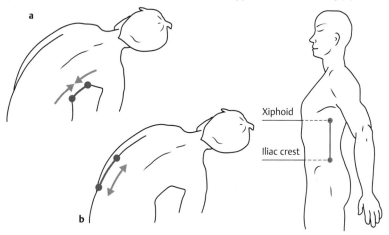

Xiphoid

Iliac crest

Measuring Thoracic Rotation with a Tape Measure

This method of measuring thoracic rotation is attributed to Pavelka (1970). It measures thoracolumbar rotation.

STEP 1 With your subject seated, measure the distance between the sternal notch and L5.

STEP 2 Ask your client to rotate and measure this distance again. Repeat with your subject rotating to the opposite direction. Note, if you are standing to the left of your subject, they should rotate to the right, as shown in the figure below.

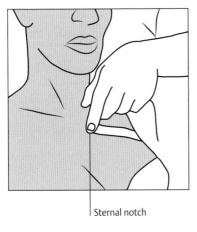

Sternal notch

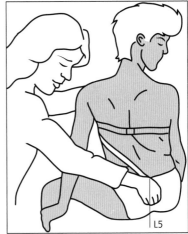

L5

Tip 10: **How to Improve Your Thoracic ROM Tape Measuring Techniques**

Question: How can I get good at measuring thoracic ROM using a tape measure?

Practice is a good way to improve a physical skill. By practicing, you will improve your skill and at the same time test the variability of using different assessment positions on the same subject, and the same test position between *different* subjects.

Ideas for improving your skill include the following:
- Use different assessment positions (sitting, standing, side lying) with the same subject.
- Assess the same movement, in the same assessment position (e.g., flexion/extension in standing) in different subjects.

- Use different bony landmarks (such as C7 and T12 or C7 and S1) with the same subject.
- Repeat the same assessment, of the same subject, over a set time period.

Look at the tables on the following pages.

Table A

This is a table you could use to record your findings for assessing flexion/extension between C7 and T12 of the same subject, using two different assessment positions, sitting and standing. (To measure extension, simply replace the column "C7–T12 in flexion" with "C7–T12 in extension.")

Table B

Alternatively, use the table B in the following pages to record your measurements for flexion in five colleagues, using one or all of the different assessment positions. The chart provided is an example of how you could record your results for thoracic flexion in five subjects in just one test position, sitting.

Table A For recording and comparing the change from neutral to flexion using C7 and T12 on the same subject in three different test positions

Assessment position		Thoracic C7–T12		
Test position	C7–T12 in neutral =	C7–T12 in flexion =	Change =
Sitting			
Standing			

Comments ....

....

....

Table B For recording and comparing the change from neutral to flexion using C7 and T12 in five subjects in sitting position

Subject	C7–T12 in neutral	C7–T12 in flexion	Difference
A			
B			
C			
D			
E			

Tip 11: **Measuring Thoracic ROM Using a Goniometer**

A goniometer is sometimes used to measure extension, lateral flexion, and rotation in the thorax and lumbar spine.

Measuring Thoracic Extension with a Goniometer: Method 1 – Standing

STEP 1 With your client standing, position the fixed arm of the goniometer vertically.

STEP 2 With your subject in extension, measure the range of motion in degrees, using the spinous process of C7 as the point with which to visually align the moving arm of your goniometer.

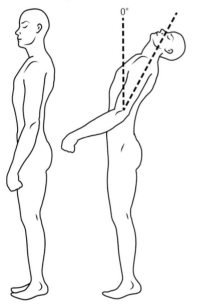

Measuring Thoracic Extension with a Goniometer: Method 2 – Prone

STEP 1 With your client prone, place the fixed arm of the goniometer horizontally.

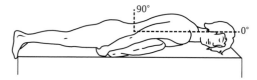

STEP 2 Ask your subject to lift their head, neck, and shoulders from the plinth and measure the range of motion in degrees, using the spinous process of C7 as the point with which to align the moving arm of your goniometer.

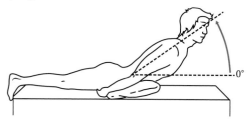

You can see that this test position, suggested in the 1965 edition of *Joint Motion, Method of Measuring and Recording*, by the American Academy of Orthopaedic Surgeons (1965), relies on the strength of spinal extensors.

An alternative would be for your subject to rest in the sphinx position.

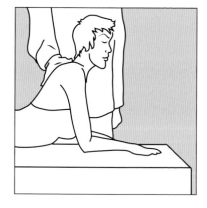

Hypermobile clients are likely to be able to extend their thoracic spines farther by pushing up through their hands and arms. In this position, the thoracic spine is extended from about T4/5 to L1.

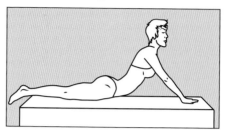

Measuring Lateral Flexion Using a Goniometer

Again, this method measures a combination of both the thoracic and lumbar spine.

STEP 1 Stand behind your subject. Position the head of the goniometer over the spinous process of S1, with one arm along the spinous processes of the spine, perpendicular to the floor.

STEP 2 Ask your client to lean to one side. Imagine a line between C7 and S1 in this position of lateral flexion and align the moving arm of your goniometer with it, pointing it toward C7. Note the angle formed between this line and the vertical spine line and take into account the curvature in the thoracic spine compared to curvature in the lumbar spine. Note any compensatory movements the client had to perform to achieve this position.

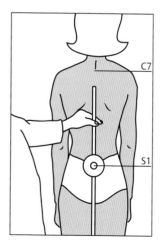

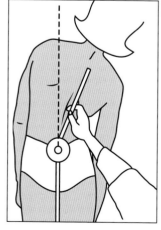

Measuring Thoracic Rotation Using a Goniometer

To minimize involvement of the neck, lumbar, and pelvic regions, it is recommended that measurement of the thoracic spine be performed with the examiner holding the subject's pelvis standing, with the subject sitting, or with the subject on their hands and knees. Unfortunately, in practice, this is difficult to achieve as you will need both of your hands to position and move the goniometer.

STEP 1 With your client seated, position the center of the goniometer over their head, with both arms of the goniometer over the acromion process on the side to which they are going to turn. The nonmoving arm of the goniometer needs to be positioned (visually) over the anterior superior iliac spines.

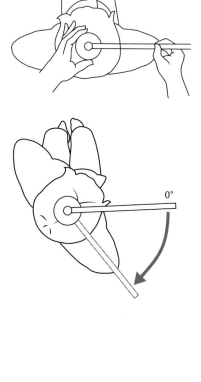

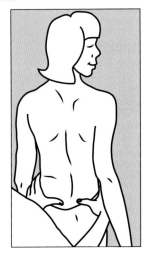

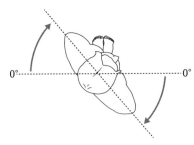

STEP 2 Ask your subject to turn their whole trunk to one side. The movable arm should follow the acromion process (on the side to which they are turning). Record your observation as the number of degrees between the stationary arm and the moving arm. Repeat to the opposite side. Note any compensatory movement.

TIP: A good trick is for your subject to rotate while holding a broom handle, which you can use to help observe rotation more easily. You can align your goniometer with the broom handle rather than with the acromion.

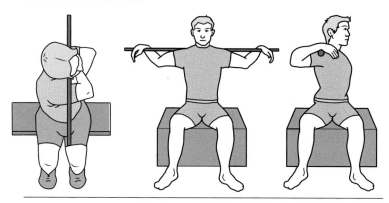

Consider in which position you are likely to get the most accurate results. Your subject may be more comfortable with their arms resting on a broom, but flexibility in their shoulder joint or tension in pectoral muscles could affect your results. Whether you choose to use a broom handle or not, you will need to stand so that you can look down on your subject and properly gauge their degree of rotation.

Question: Does it matter if my subject flexes when rotating?

Yes, it is important that your subject sits up straight when they perform the test as the results are different if they rotate while their trunk is flexed.

As an interesting exercise, you could partner with two fellow students or colleagues and record your thoracic rotation with and without pelvic stabilization.

Full descriptions of how to use a goniometer are to be found in Norkin and White (1985).

Subject	Rotation in degrees without pelvic stabilization		Rotation in degrees with pelvic stabilization	
	Left	Right	Left	Right
A				
B				
C				

Tip 12: How Can I Tell What Is a Normal Thoracic ROM?

The American Academy of Orthopaedic Surgeons (1965) suggested that when measuring from C7 to S1 there is an increase of 4 in (10.2 cm) in total spinal flexion: 1 in (2.5 cm) in the thoracic spine and 3 in (7.6 cm) in the lumbar spine.

In extension there is in an overall decrease of 1.6 in (4 cm): 0.4 in (1 cm) from thoracic and 1.2 in (3 cm) from lumbar.

As you can see, when you discover an increase or a decrease in a measurement when using a tape measure to measure the distance between C7 and S1, it is difficult to say precisely from which part of the spine this increase/decrease originates.

In their study assessing ROM using a tape measure, Moll and Wright (1971) remind us that it is important to remember that while spinal ROM decreases with age, within each age category there is wide variance in abilities and therefore in ROM findings.

Range of movement when using a tape measure

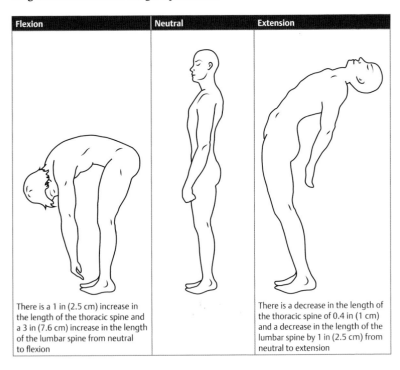

Flexion	Neutral	Extension
There is a 1 in (2.5 cm) increase in the length of the thoracic spine and a 3 in (7.6 cm) increase in the length of the lumbar spine from neutral to flexion		There is a decrease in the length of the thoracic spine of 0.4 in (1 cm) and a decrease in the length of the lumbar spine by 1 in (2.5 cm) from neutral to extension

Range of movement when using a goniometer

Range of movement	Neutral position	Example
Flexion Normal = 80–90 degrees in standing		
Extension Normal = 20–30 degrees from neutral in standing (approximately 20 degrees from neutral in prone)		
Lateral flexion Normal = 20–35 degrees from neutral		

| Rotation

Normal = 30–45 degrees from neutral | 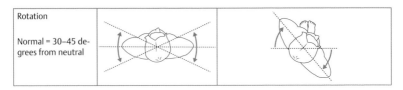 |

Previous sections contain charts showing normal ROMs for the thoracic spine: ROM in inches (and centimeters) when measuring ROM using a tape measure (p. 186) compared to ROM measured in degrees using a goniometer (pp. 187–188). Your own measurements will no doubt reveal variations between individuals, with ROM findings changing due to age, injury, and illness, as well as the way we use our bodies. Measurement findings are often reported differently between studies. One explanation for the variance in findings is that in some studies, measurements were taken with the subjects standing, whereas in others the subjects were seated; in some studies, the movements were performed actively; in others, they were performed passively. Different methods give different results. The figures provided in this *tip* can therefore only be a rough guide. Making ROM measurements regularly will help you to gain an understanding of normal parameters for your individual clients. Knowing those parameters can help you determine whether your interventions have been successful in improving ROM, and can help identify when your client has been doing something that might have contributed to a decrease in ROM.

For further details, see Greene and Heckman (1994).

Tip 13: **Documenting Thoracic Range of Movement**

There are many different ways to document ROM. One method is to use a set pattern of lines onto which you record your findings. The end of each line represents full ROM.

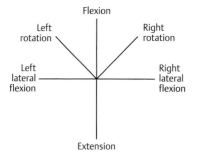

Placing a cross or dash over any of these lines can be used to record your observations. On the next page are some hypothetical examples of three different subjects together with information about their thoracic ROM, and an accompanying sketch to indicate how these observations might be recorded.

For example, the following findings would be recorded like this:

Example A
- Flexion: reduced by 75%.
- Extension: reduced by 75%.
- Right rotation: reduced by 25%.
- Left rotation: reduced by 25%.
- Right lateral flexion: reduced by 75%.
- Left lateral flexion: reduced by 75%.

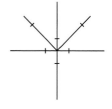

Example B
- Flexion: full/normal.
- Extension: full/normal.
- Right rotation: full/normal.
- Left rotation: reduced by 50%.
- Right lateral flexion: full/normal.
- Left lateral flexion: reduced by 50%.

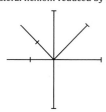

Example C
- Flexion: greater than normal.
- Extension: greater than normal.
- Right rotation: greater than normal.
- Left rotation: greater than normal.
- Right lateral flexion: greater than normal.
- Left lateral flexion: greater than normal.

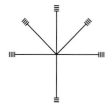

Tip 14: Assessing Thoracic Excursion Using Palpation

Standing behind your seated subject, place your hands gently on their back, cupping the lower ribs and with your thumbs approximately over the spinous process of the T10. As your client breathes in and out at their normal rate, observe your thumbs and notice whether these move equidistantly from the spine. Asymmetry could indicate a restriction in the intercostals on that side.

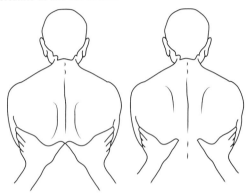

Question: Do I need to assess my client in a standing position?

No, you may find this easier if the subject is sitting on a raised plinth and you are sitting on a chair behind them, or even kneeling. An alternative position in which to assess your subject is to ask them to straddle a chair while you kneel behind them.

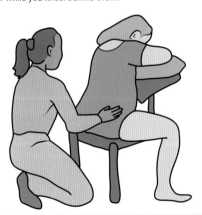

TIP: Breathing patterns change depending on the position of your client. Compare rib excursion with your subject in different test positions: standing, sitting, or sitting with the arms supported as if resting on the steering wheel of a car. Use the table below to record your findings. Do you notice any differences?

Position	Findings
Sitting	
Standing	
Driving	

TIP: When assessing a client with a history of shoulder dysfunction, rib asymmetry is often discovered on the side of the dysfunction.

TIP: If you gently place your hands on your client's shoulders while they are breathing normally, you can identify whether "accessory" muscles of respiration are working harder than normal, as this is felt as elevation of the shoulder during inhalation. Do both shoulders raise and lower to the same extent as your subject inhales and exhales? What are your findings when you assess a subject with a shoulder injury?

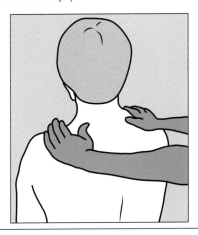

Note: Any muscle attached to a rib is a muscle that facilitates breathing. The so-called accessory muscles have a significant part to play in breathing mechanics and while they are termed "accessory," they should not be considered insignificant.

191

Tip 15: Assessing Thoracic Excursion Using a Tape Measure

Being able to measure thoracic expansion is important as it helps to determine change in subjects with conditions affecting the rib cage, such as ankylosing spondylitis. Being able to take baseline measurements of a client's ability to expand their rib cage helps determine the effectiveness of interventions designed to improve the function of vertebral and costovertebral joints and muscles affecting inspiration and expiration. A good article on this subject is that by Bockenhauer et al (2007). You will need to take readings at two different positions:

- *For upper thoracic expansion*, beneath the axilla.
- *For lower thoracic expansion*, the T10 rib level.

Upper thoracic	Lower thoracic
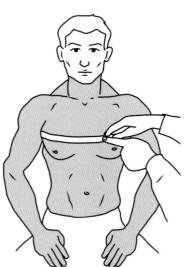	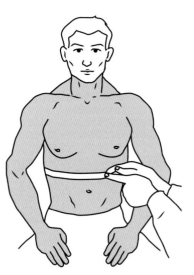

Using either of the positions shown above, take the following steps:

STEP 1 Take your first measurement when the subject has exhaled.

STEP 2 Take your second measurement when they have inhaled. Calculate the difference in readings to determine the number of inches (or centimeters) by which the subject can expand their rib cage.

Use the following table as a guide to how you could record your findings. Normal expansion is approximately 1 to 3 in (3–8 cm). How do your findings compare with these figures?

Table to show results of thoracic excursion measurements for three different subjects

A	Expiration	Inspiration	Difference
Upper thorax			
Lower thorax			

B	Expiration	Inspiration	Difference
Upper thorax			
Lower thorax			

C	Expiration	Inspiration	Difference
Upper thorax			
Lower thorax			

Subjects with altered breathing patterns often have pain on excursion. Reduced excursion can help identify that a subject may have one or more hypomobile ribs.

TIP: You could even take a midthoracic reading if you wanted, at the nipple line.

Tip 16: Assessing Thoracic "Stiffness"

Do you ever come across clients who feel that they need to self-release their thorax—clients who perform movements to "crack" themselves, often on a regular basis? If so, this *tip* may be of particular interest to you.

Any book about the thorax would not be complete without mention of Lee (2006, 2008) and the superb contribution she has made to our understanding of this part of the body. Just a small sample of her suggestions for thoracic assessment are included here, selected on the basis that they are suitable for massage therapists—who usually have exceptional skills of palpation—and student sports therapists, physiotherapists, osteopaths, and chiropractors whose job it is to make assessments regarding biomechanic dysfunction.

Lee argues that for the thorax to function optimally a person must have correct control of thoracic "rings." She describes a ring as consisting of an intervertebral disk, the two vertebrae immediately adjacent to it, and the ribs associated with those two vertebrae, including their attachment to the sternum anteriorly.

Lee postulates that the increased resting tone in global muscles compresses segments of the spine, and this is sometimes misinterpreted by clinicians as articular stiffness. The increase in tone of global muscles may be compensatory for the *decrease* in tone in specific parts of some of the deeper muscles responsible for segmental control of the spine, namely, thoracic multifidus, the intercostals, the levator costarum, and the diaphragm.

The full thoracic assessment procedures suggested by Lee are beyond the scope of this book, but to give you an appreciation of her ideas, try these simple assessment tests based on her recommendations for improvements in thoracic examination.

Assessment Test 1: Increased or Decreased Activity in Longissimus on Trunk Rotation

During rotation of the trunk to the left, for example, there is decreased activity in the longissimus muscle on the right in a subject who is pain free. However, Lee has found that, when performing this same movement, palpation reveals there is often *increased* activity in the right longissimus muscle in subjects with thoracic pain.

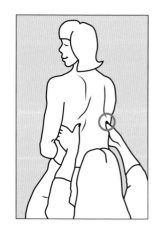

Ask your client to sit on a stool, their feet comfortably placed on the floor. Palpate longissimus as your client rotates to the left. Do you notice an increase or a decrease in the contralateral muscle? Repeat, asking your subject to rotate to the right.

You could use the chart below to record your findings on testing six subjects, three symptomatic and three asymptomatic, using an arrow to show whether there is an *increase* or a *decrease* in tone in the contralateral muscle.

	Symptomatic subjects			Asymptomatic subjects		
	1	2	3	1	2	3
On rotation of the thorax to the *right*: increase or decrease in activation of longissimus on the *left* of the spine?						
On rotation of the thorax to the *left*: increase or decrease in activation of longissimus on the *right* of the spine?						

Do you agree with Lee that on rotation there is an increase in activation in the contralateral longissumus muscle in subjects with thoracic pain? Did you find that there is a decrease in activation in longissimus in subjects who are pain free?

Assessment Test 2: Sitting Arm Lift as an Indication of Loss of Thoracic "Ring" Control

Lee explains that the thorax should provide a stable base during initiation of shoulder flexion, and on initiation of flexion there should be *no* activation in the contralateral longissimus muscle in healthy subjects. Try this assessment for yourself, comparing subjects who are asymptomatic with subjects with thoracic symptoms.

Standing behind your subject, ask them to take their arm slowly above their head. As your subject initiates the movement, do you feel anything in their longissimus muscle?

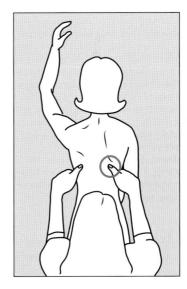

Assessment Test 3: Palpating Multifidus

Lee describes how multifidus may be found to have a decrease in resting tone, or may even have atrophied, in those segments of

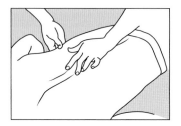

the spine that are not functioning optimally. Test this by palpating a subject with thoracic pain.

Further, Lee states that when the muscle is palpated during specific tasks, it is revealed to lack recruitment in symptomatic subjects. With your subject in the prone position, ask them to abduct their arm while you palpate multifidus. Whether you are simply palpating, or palpating while your subject moves their arm, compare your findings when applying these tests to a subject without thoracic pain. Do you discover any differences?

Assessment Test 4: The Rib Cage Wiggle

Lee (2006) proposes this test to reveal the amount of rigidity in the superficial muscles connecting the thorax and pelvis. With your client standing or supine, place one of your hands on the lateral aspect of their rib cage on one side of their body and your other hand on the lateral aspect of their pelvis on the other side of their body and simultaneously apply gentle pressure. Do this several times in a gentle, oscillatory movement, observing how much force is required. There should be a "wiggle." Reverse your hands and "wiggle" your subject in the opposite direction. If it is not possible to elicit the "wiggle," this indicates rigidity and excessive muscle activity, especially when this is observed in a supine subject, supposedly relaxed.

(Interestingly, this shearing type test is similar to a myofascial release treatment that requires the same movement to be encouraged, but for a different reason.)

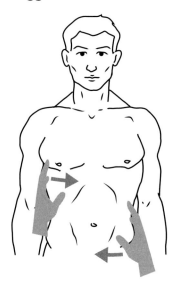

Tip 17: **Identifying Thoracic Subluxations**

Muscles such as semispinalis, multifidus, and rotatores can bring about a rotation in vertebrae when opposing muscles are weak or paralysed. To identify such rotations, Maitland (2001) suggests palpating the spine with a subject seated, feeling the transverse processes of each vertebra, with your thumbs. When you feel a protrusion beneath your thumb, this is a rotated vertebra and the side of the protrusion is the side to which the vertebra is rotated. For example, if you feel that the transverse process of a vertebra is more prominent on the left, then that is the side to which the vertebra is rotated, as the bone has moved toward you (a). You should feel a corresponding indentation on the opposite side of the spine, formed by the position of the transverse process away from you (b).

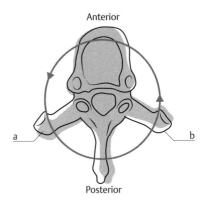

Anterior

a

b

Posterior

TIP: Maitland suggests that when you are learning, you focus only on those vertebrae that seem most prominent and to leave any about which you are unsure. As you become more proficient in your palpation skills, you will become more adept at locating subluxed vertebrae and will know to which side they are rotated.

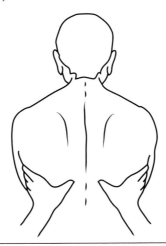

Rose (2008) suggests an alternative approach: with your subject adopting a position of lateral flexion while in the prone position. Try to avoid your subject rotating their thorax. Next, palpate the spinous processes. Rose says that these should follow the natural curve created by lateral flexion of the spine (a) while in this position. Those spinous processes which do not follow the natural curve are subluxed (b).

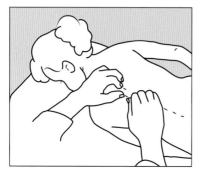

Rose describes another three ways to assess the thorax that reveal clues to regions you may wish to investigate further.

Experiment with Rose's suggestions and decide for yourself on their value.

Method 1

Brush your fingers rapidly up and down either side of the thoracic spine, keeping your touch light. Increased perspiration in regions of abnormality will prevent the smooth flow of your fingers over the skin.

Method 2

Scratch lightly all over the back in a vigorous manner and then watch as erethyma develops. Rose says that the area that stays reddest the longest will be at the same level and on the same side as the "blocked" joint.

Method 3

Palpate the spinous processes of each vertebra. Swelling or thickening indicates a "stuck" joint.

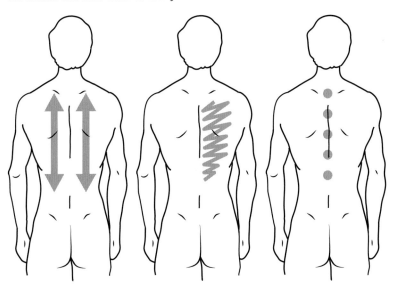

Tip 18: Quick Tests for Pectoral Length

Shortness in pectoral muscles contributes to muscle imbalance and impairs the proper functioning of the thorax.

Six different methods for assessing shortness in pectorals are discussed in the following sections. Each method is quick and simple.

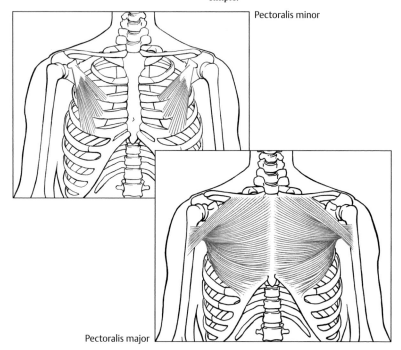

Pectoralis minor

Pectoralis major

Method 1

One of the easiest methods to assess for pectoral shortness is simply to ask your subject to lie supine and observe the position of their shoulders. Both shoulders should rest against the plinth/treatment couch (a). If one shoulder appears higher (b) off the couch than the other, one explanation is shortness in pectoralis minor on that side.

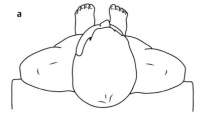

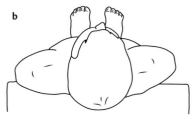

If the goal of your treatment was to lengthen these muscles, you could even measure the position of the shoulders, choosing a common bony landmark, and then measure again after your intervention.

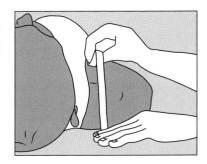

Method 2

A second way to assess the muscles is to apply gentle pressure to the head of the humerus, pressing gently toward the couch. A decrease in movement could indicate shortness in the pectorals on that side.

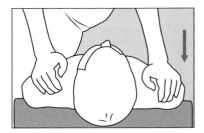

Question: Is this a safe test for all of my clients?

Caution is needed when assessing clients with rheumatoid arthritis and other known conditions affecting their shoulder joint, as translation of the humeral head in this test could be aggravating.

TIP: Press one side at a time and compare the left shoulder to the right.

Method 3

This method helps assess the length of pectoralis major. With your subject supine, their arms should rest on the couch with elbows pointing outward (a). An elbow that is raised (b) suggests shortness in the pectorals on that side.

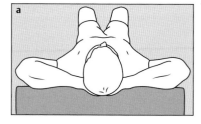
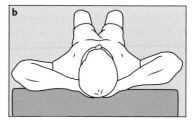

Method 4

A fourth way to assess pectorals is to compare left and right sides of the chest, measuring from the sternal notch (a) to the coracoid process (b). Measurements should be the same on both left and right sides. Where a measurement is less on one side, this indicates protraction of the shoulder on that side and a shortening of pectoralis minor on that side.

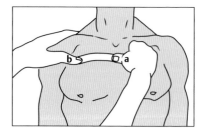

Method 5

Ask your subject to perform horizontal extension, taking the arms behind them and to report back as to which side feels most "tight."

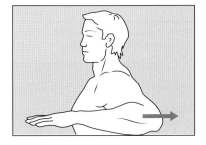

TIP: A common mistake is to ask the client to extend their shoulder with the elbow extended. This tensions tissues of the arm and forearm and if these are tight, it can give a false reading, indicating pectorals are shortened when they are not.

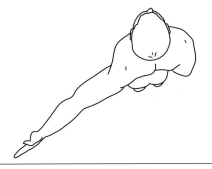

Method 6

Taking the arms into elevation, in either the supine or standing position, tests the length of latissimus dorsi and teres major. Arms should rest overhead on a couch or wall (a). If they do not (b), this indicates muscle shortness.

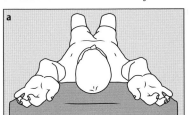
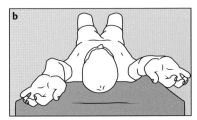

TIP: Remember that performing the test in a standing position also tests the strength of muscles to flex and elevate the shoulder.

TIP: You could choose to measure the distance of the subject's hand from a wall or couch, depending on your initial test position, before and after treatment.

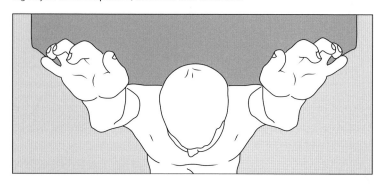

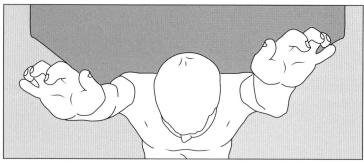

Note that the flexibility of your subject's elbow and wrist joints will affect this test because you are measuring the distance of the hand (or wrist) from the wall or couch.

Tip 19: Appreciating Erector Spinae

This muscle group is responsible for keeping the vertebral column erect, working concentrically to raise the trunk from a flexed position, isometrically to maintain a neutral or flexed position, and eccentrically in trunk flexion. Maintaining any one of these positions—unsupported forward flexion, a static sitting or standing posture, or extension—is likely to fatigue these muscles.

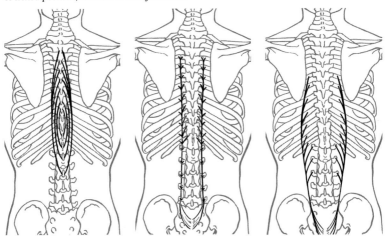

Further, with an increase in the kyphotic curve associated with poor posture, these muscles are lengthened, weakened, and unable to function optimally.

TIP: It is important when assessing that we palpate with a client in the prone position; otherwise, we are attempting to palpate muscles that are actively engaged in trying to keep the vertebral column erect. Palpating a person as they sit or stand is likely to reveal an increase in tone in these muscles, something which one would expect when palpating an active muscle. In the prone position, the subject can relax and we can feel for abnormalities in tone.

Have you ever come across a client who complains of back pain and on palpation you find the erector spinae to be hypersensitive and with a palpable increase in tone, aggravated by light touch? We need to ask "why do muscles usually spasm?" and to remember that one reason they spasm is as a response to injury to adjacent structures. If you suspect injury to structures associated with erector spinae, will relaxing these muscles be helpful or unhelpful? In some cases, muscles continue to spasm after the original injury is resolved. Where pain results from the spasm itself, reduction in the spasm will be helpful. Where there is an ongoing, underlying problem with a joint, relaxation of a spasming erector spinae muscle is unlikely to last: as soon as your client tries to move from prone, muscles will fire and respasm protectively.

Tip 20: **Cloward's Points**

In his fascinating article of 1959, Cloward noted that cervical disks could be responsible for referring pain to other structures of the body. One of these regions was the medial border of the scapula. If you are struggling to resolve a symptom in the rhomboid region, consider leaving the thorax and turning your attention to your client's cervical spine. Assess this region for hypertonicity and note any previous trauma. Could this be the cause of your client's symptoms? Note that rib dysfunction can also produce pain along the medial border of the scapula. Consider using Tip 22: Assessing Ribs (pp. 209–210).

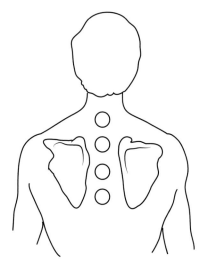

Tip 21: **The Rhomboid Myth**

Therapists are getting wise to the fact that if they are treating a client with "poor" posture, characterized by a slumped thorax and protracted shoulders, the rhomboid muscles—in a region in which many clients report intense pain—are in a lengthened position, not a shortened position. In such subjects, pectoralis minor and tissues of the anterior chest wall are shortened and weak, while rhomboids (and erector spinae) are lengthened and weak. This has implications for how we treat clients with kyphotic postures.

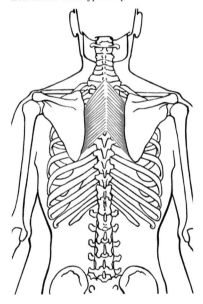

Therapists frequently report feeling "knots" in rhomboid muscles. So what are these?

There are several explanations for firm, palpable areas in the region of the rhomboids:

- Normal muscle anatomy.
- Normal bony anatomy.
- Trigger points.
- Cloward's points.
- Scar tissue.
- Lipomas.
- Serious pathology.

Normal muscle anatomy: The fibers of the middle portion of the trapezius muscle, the fibers of rhomboid muscles, and the fibers of erector spinae muscles all run in different directions. These muscles cross, and are adhered to one another. Might an area of increased tone be nothing more than normal muscle anatomy? How would we know? When there is a localized area of unusually high tone, this would be tender on compression if it were a trigger point, and painless in most cases if the spot in question is a lipoma or scar tissue.

Normal bony anatomy: It could be that the region you are palpating is the normal angle of a rib, which happens to be particularly prominent in that subject. Again, in the absence of unusual pathology this would be painless on compression.

Trigger points: These are localized points of tenderness that are painful on light compression and where the pain dissipates within a short period of time, perhaps within a minute. If the pain does not dissipate, this is unlikely to be a trigger point and the point should not be compressed.

Cloward's points: These are areas of pain referred from the cervical spine to the medial border of the scapulae, described by Cloward in 1959 (see Tip 20, p. 206, for more information). However, such points may be painful, but they are not necessarily palpable, as the source of the pain is the neck.

Scar tissue: Unless there is an acute injury, scar tissue is painless on compression.

However, tearing of the fibers of rhomboids is not common and your client must have been engaged in an activity where the rhomboids were either suddenly overstretched, forced into contraction, or compressed to such a degree as to cause tearing.

Lipomas: These are fatty nodules, painless on compression.

Serious pathology: You may palpate a region that a client reports as being extremely painful and in rare cases this can indicate serious pathology. This could be a herniated disk, prior to which the client will usually have suffered a traumatic event, or it could indicate cancer in a thoracic vertebra. In either case, you should not treat this client but refer them back to their doctor. Herniations of disks within the thoracic spine are rare; so is cancer in this region without there having been a history of this disease. As manual therapists, we are well placed to help identify potentially serious conditions that manifest as painful lumps in the thoracic region and should always refer if in doubt as to any condition we are treating.

Tip 22: Assessing Ribs

Ribs articulate with thoracic vertebrae and, therefore affect, and are affected by this region of the spine. The radiate ligament at the head of each rib connects with the bodies of two vertebrae and the intervertebral disk between them. Some very simple ways to assess ribs are described here. If you are reading this as a student of physical therapy, osteopathy, or chiropractic, you are likely to learn many more techniques. If you are reading this as a massage therapist or sports therapist, the assessments described here may be new to you and could help with assessing clients who come to you complaining of back pain. The assessments should be used in conjunction with Tips 14 and 15: Assessing Thoracic Excursion (pp. 190–191 and 192–193).

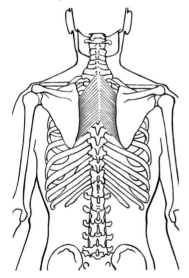

Assessment 1 Ask your subject to place their arms across their chest and observe them posteriorly. Look for the contour of the ribs on each side. Do rib contours appear normal or do any stand out? Do ribs appear symmetrical? Are any rib angles particularly prominent?

Assessment 2 Run the flat of your hand over your subject's back. Do any ribs feel prominent?

Assessment 3 With your subject prone, palpate their ribs as they breathe normally. Place the fingertips of one hand on a rib on the right side of their body and the fingertips of your other hand on a rib on the left side of the body and compare how each rib moves. Work your way up or down the thorax assessing ribs simultaneously left and right at each level of the spine.

Assessment 4 With your subject in the prone position apply gentle pressure to the ribs to assess their "spring." One at a time, using your thenar eminence over each rib angle, apply gentle pressure and then suddenly release. "Free" ribs "spring" back; "fixed" or "stuck" ribs do not. *This is contraindicated in acute conditions or in subjects suffering rheumatoid conditions or osteoporosis. In subjects with ankylosing spondylitis, ribs may be fused with no spring discernible at all. Obviously you would not do this assessment where a client has an acute condition.*

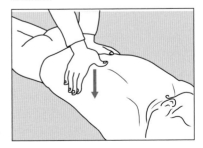

Question: How do I know which rib I am on?

The angle of the 8th rib is most deviated from the midline, so it is sometimes more easy to palpate than rib angles. You can then lightly locate a rib angle more medial, both above (the 7th rib) and below (the 9th rib). The only way to be really certain which rib you are on is to count down from the 1st rib (palpable beneath the upper fibers of trapezius and frequently very painful in subjects) or up from the 12th and 11th ribs.

The Relationship between Ribs and Vertebrae

When the body of a thoracic vertebra rotates counterclockwise, to the left, if you are standing behind your subject, its spinous process moves counterclockwise also, to the right. The ribs, attached to the vertebrae, also move: they become convex on the anterior, right side of the body, and also convex on the posterior, left side of the body.

Your observations of rib position could therefore give you clues as to the position of the accompanying vertebra and the direction to which it is rotated; your observations of the spinous processes of the thoracic vertebrae give you clues to the position of ribs.

Become convex

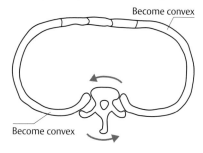

Become convex

Tip 23: Assessing Vertebral Restrictions – Subjective

This assessment is safe but unorthodox. It takes about 5 minutes and requires a quiet room. It is likely to suit some clients but not others. Some therapists may find it unappealing, while others may be curious to experiment with its usefulness. Based on subjective feedback, it can be useful in helping to identify regions of the spine where there may be restrictions, such as facet joint impactions or subluxations, where the client has previously struggled to describe their symptoms or to identify a specific anatomical location for their problem.

It is helpful if you have a model of a spine you can show to your client before you begin this assessment, so that they can see the three groups of vertebrae: cervical, thoracic, and lumbar. You do not have to use those words; you could describe the bones as "neck," "upper back," and "lower back."

You do not need to observe your client and so could read from a script you have written as your subject rests in the prone position.

Example of a script for use while assessing vertebral restrictions:

Breathe normally. Allow yourself to relax. As you relax, imagine that the air you are breathing can flow into your spine. Notice what happens as you breathe in, and imagine the air flowing into the bones of your neck. Breathe in and out as normal. Notice what happens to the air as it flows into the bones of your upper back and ribs. Breathe in and out as normal. Finally, notice what happens to the air as it flows down into the bones of your lower back. And as you continue to breathe in and out: the air flows into your neck, and upper back, and lower back. Ask yourself how

that feels. Does the air flow in freely or are there any restrictions? Does the air feel smooth and flowing, or does it have some other quality? Is the air clear or colored? Does the air have a vibrational quality to it? Does the air flow through all of the bones of your spine in the same way? Are there any areas that feel restricted or different? Does it flow in and out at the same pace? Continue to breathe normally, noting the air and its qualities as it flows through your neck, upper back, and lower back. When you are ready, open your eyes and take a few moments before sitting up.

When your client is sitting up and ready, ask them to report back to you anything they noted during this assessment. They may have nothing to report, or they may have identified areas where the passage of air felt blocked or that it vibrated differently, or that it even changed color.

The rationale behind this assessment technique for soliciting subjective feedback is that when a person is given the opportunity to relax in a guided way and in an environment in which they feel safe, they are more likely to be able to identify regions of their spine that feel different. As a therapist, you can then use this information to explore those regions with further assessment, should you wish to.

Although this is an example of a non-evidence-based assessment, appropriate only for some clients, and for use where a therapist has the time to facilitate such a slow assessment, it gives the client the opportunity to try and pinpoint the problem region in their spine while in the safe environment of a therapist's treatment room.

Tip 24: Assessing Soft Tissue Restrictions with Palpation

Here are four simple tips to aid your palpation.

First, work methodically, as opposed to in a random manner. As if mowing a lawn, palpate horizontally, left to right, or vertically up and down, on one side of the body. Then repeat on

the opposite side. In this way, you are certain to cover the entire area in question.

Second, practice with different methods of palpation. For example, gentle gripping (a) or fingertip traction (b) to help determine the pliability of tissues.

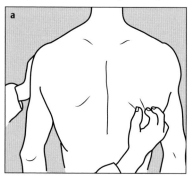

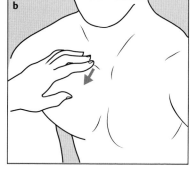

Third, push (or drag!) tissues north, east, south, and west in order to determine their pliability, comparing one side of the body with the other.

Fourth, compare how the tissues feel when your subject is standing with how the tissues feel when they are sitting or in lying positions. Use this table as an example.

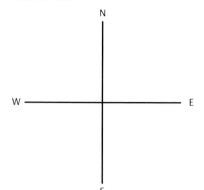

	Standing	Sitting	Prone or supine
Rhomboids			
Upper pectoral fibers			
Latissimus dorsi			

Tip 25: **Assessment of Superficial Fascia**

Restrictions in superficial fascia may be determined by placing the palm of your hand flat against the skin and, keeping it pressed against the skin, moving the skin in different directions, as you assess for pliability.

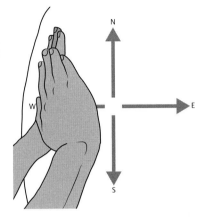

TIP: One way to think of this is as a north-east–south-west assessment.

You can assess tissues of the anterior thorax in the same manner.

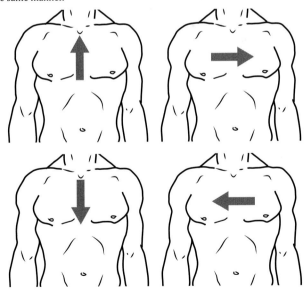

Tip 26: Back Assessment – An Eastern Approach

In *Step-by-Step Shiatsu* by Ohashi (1977), a statement (on prelim p. vi) reads, "In order to help achieve a healthy world the author would like to share his knowledge with the West." It seems fitting to end this chapter with two techniques based on Ohashi's descriptions because, whether an experienced practitioner such as Ohashi, or a newly qualified or even student therapist, we all have something to contribute to the world of therapy, no matter what our training or philosophy.

Using Your Palm

With your subject in the prone position, place your palm directly over their spine, so that your fingers are parallel with the spine, with your middle finger over the spine itself.

Using gentle pressure, work from the top of the spine to its base. Ohashi says that using this technique you will be able to identify stiffness and areas of muscle spasm.

Sliding Diagnosis

With your subject seated, ask them to bend forward, flexing their spine so that the spinous processes become accentuated. Using firm pressure, slide the fingertips of your middle and index fingers down the spine.

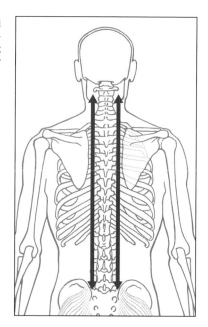

Question: Does it matter whether I slide my fingers from the neck to the sacrum or from the sacrum to the neck?

No. Ohashi suggests that you slide from the neck down if you are standing behind your client and from the base of the spine upward if you are standing in front of your client.

Chapter V

Thoracic Treatment

Chapter 5 **Thoracic Treatment**

Have you ever felt that as a massage thera-pist you are delivering the same form of back treatments over and over again? You may be treating your clients individually and ac-knowledging their subjective feedback, yet the hands-on treatment you provide varies little among clients. Many therapists report to me that over the years they have begun to feel a little "stale," wanting to vary their treatments but at the same time being cau-tious as to whether other techniques will be as effective.

Provided here are a large selection of tips, techniques which I have found helpful in breaking up the monotony of a regular tho-racic massage treatment. Of course, they should be used with a specific purpose in mind. This might be to relax a client, to reduce stiffness globally or locally, to stretch muscles, or to lengthen soft tissues. As with all the tips in this book, it is use-ful to experiment, not only in trialing the

techniques, but also in receiving them. So much can be learned from experiencing how a technique feels, so I encourage you to be the "client" for one of your colleagues and to work together to explore these suggestions.

There are a few clients for whom the tips provided here are contraindicated. You may already know that unexplained pain in a lo-calized area of the thorax is a warning sign, so clients presenting in this way should be referred to a doctor. Most of the tips provid-ed here can be applied to most clients. There are some that are for specific client groups, such as those with "flat back," in the thorac-ic region, or an exaggerated kyphosis. When working with clients, ask yourself what is it that you are hoping to achieve, and then whether the suggested tip fits that purpose. After practicing with a colleague, ask which of these treatments you enjoyed receiving yourself.

Tip 1: How Thought Affects Muscle Tone

Have you ever used stretching or massage to reduce the tone in muscles? Unless you are using tapotement techniques, massage is most often used to relax soft tissues and bring about a decrease in their tone. It is therefore important to find ways to facilitate this and to avoid situations during the treatment where tone may become elevated. There are two interesting experiments you can do to demonstrate how thought affects muscle tone.

Experiment 1

With your subject in the prone position, feel for the rhomboid muscles. Ask your subject to contract their rhomboids, drawing their scapulae toward the spine. Both you and your subject can feel these muscles contracting and you can observe the scapulae change position. Now that your subject knows which muscles you want them to focus on, ask them to see if they can contract these muscles without moving their scapulae. As you continue to palpate, you will feel the muscles contract simply as a result of the client thinking about drawing their scapulae back toward their spine.

Experiment 2

A second experiment you can try works best if you use someone who engages regularly in a sporting activity, especially if this involves a lot of upper limb action such as racket sports, throwing, rowing, or climbing. With your subject lying comfortably in the prone position, place your hands gently on the muscles of their thorax. Ask your subject not to talk to you. Once you feel that your client is comfortable and has relaxed, ask them to think about performing their particular sport in a way that makes them feel energized and excited. Perhaps they might envisage reaching to hit or to shoot a ball, swimming extra fast, or pulling themselves up a rock face. As your client engages in thinking about their activity, you will notice an increase in tone in the muscles beneath your hands.

These two simple experiments have been included as a treatment tip—rather than as an assessment tip—because they demonstrate that it can be disadvantageous to engage a client in conversation if your purpose is to decrease tone, perhaps through massage or stretching. This is especially true if your conversation involves them thinking about their own particular physical activity.

Tip 2: Encouraging Thoracic Expansion

You may wish to encourage thoracic expansion:

- When treating a client in the post-acute stage following intercostal strain or a rib fracture, where they are likely to have maintained a hunched, protective posture.
- When working with asthmatic clients.
- When trying to encourage clients to have a greater awareness of their bodies for the purposes of postural correction.
- When working with a client who is prone to maintaining a hunched posture at work or when engaged in a hobby.
- To facilitate an initial stretch in soft tissues of the thorax when treating clients in the post-acute stages following operations such as mastectomy.
- To help calm those clients prone to anxiety.

This tip explains how a therapist can facilitate thoracic expansion in a safe manner. You may wish to assess thoracic expansion before and after this technique, using either Tip 14 (pp. 255–258) or Tip 15 (pp. 259–261) in Chapter 4.

STEP 1 Position your client so that they are comfortably seated, straddling a chair, perhaps with a pillow against their chest and stomach, or in the prone position. They may be fully clothed as long as they are comfortable. Sit or kneel behind them and place your hands on their back, spreading your fingers to "cup" the posterolateral ribs, and with your palms flat against your client's body. Apply firm but gentle pressure through your palms. Encourage your client to breathe normally. Feel the movement as their rib cage expands and contracts with inhalation.

STEP 2 As your client inhales, ever so slightly decrease your hand pressure. With their next inspiration, your subject will increase their inspiration, expanding their rib cage as they naturally try to breathe "into" your palms.

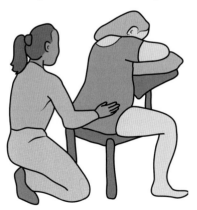

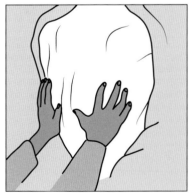

Question: Can this technique be performed with my client on a couch?

Yes, with your client in the prone position, stand at the head of the couch and reach over to place your hands on the lower ribs. Notice that you cannot apply pressure in quite the same way in this position as when you treat a seated client. With the client supine or in a semi-reclined position you can access the inferior ribs, but notice that to do so you need to maintain a position in which you are flexed at the waist, and this could harm your own back.

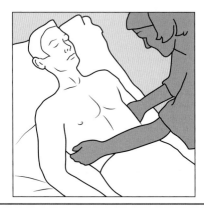

During different sessions, you could compare the difference between the following:
- Different treatment positions.
- The same position but different hand placements.
- Performing this technique with or without a verbal prompt.

An example of a prompt is, "Try to keep your chest wall touching my hands as you breathe in."

Question: How many times can this technique be performed?

Once your client is relaxed, avoid asking them to inhale more than three times in order to prevent hyperventilation.

There are many exercises that a client may do for themselves to help expand their rib cage, some of which are described in Chapter 6, Tip 5: Breathing Exercises (pp. 306–309).

Tip 3: Rocking Spinous Processes

This technique is particularly useful:

- When working with clients with a reduced range of movement in the thorax.
- When treating clients who report their upper back feeling "stiff."
- Where you feel thoracic segments are palpably "stuck."
- When treating hypermobile clients who may have tension in localized segments of the thorax.

This technique affects the joints of the thorax by bringing about a minor stretch in the soft tissues associated with these joints—including costovertebral joints—as each individual thoracic vertebra is rotated to a minor degree. It is not appropriate for clients with osteoporosis or fused joints, and would be unhelpful if applied to segments of the spine that are hypermobile. Obviously it should not be used in acute conditions of any kind, including herniations. Given the gentle nature of the technique, it is unlikely to be harmful if used when treating clients

with scoliosis. However, given the complex nature of the scoliotic spine, it would be unwise to use the technique with the intention of bringing about anatomical change. It could, however, be beneficial in treating clients with scoliosis, where your goal is a decrease in muscle tone, or when treating clients with thoracic pain that you believe is of muscular origin.

STEP 1 With your client in the prone position, stand to one side of the treatment couch. Locate the spinous processes of the thoracic spine and position your thumbs, reinforced as shown, against the side of one of the processes. Keep the flat pad of your thumb against the process rather than the tip of your thumb. You would not usually be encouraged to press through a thumb joint in this way, but this pressure is very slight, and reinforcing your thumbs as pictured reduces the likelihood of injury to your own joints.

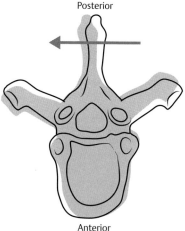

Posterior

Anterior

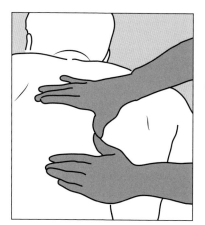

Question: Does it matter where I start the rocking, at the superior or inferior thoracic region?

No, you can start wherever it feels appropriate. It is good to be consistent, however, because you will need to document your findings: does the client report discomfort when you "rock" a particular vertebra or does a particular section of the thorax feel less able (or more able) to rock than other areas? Such findings indicate hypomobility or hypermobility of that segment.

STEP 2 Using gentle pressure, push the spinous process away from you using a gentle rocking motion, one, two, or three times. Work your way down the spine and then move to the opposite side of the couch and repeat on the other side of the spine.

The purpose of your "rocking" is to help relax soft tissues and decrease pressure on joints. Do not force any vertebrae which feel stuck: this is not a manipulative technique. If one segment feels less mobile than the others, leave it and return to it later. You may have already discovered that the body sometimes responds better to gentle, subtle techniques than to forcible ones.

TIP: One way to think of this technique is to imagine the spinous processes are like a sail on a sailboat and you are facilitating a tilting motion. Of course, the spinous processes in the thoracic region are not as prominent as a sail on a sailboat, as they lie flatter to the spine.

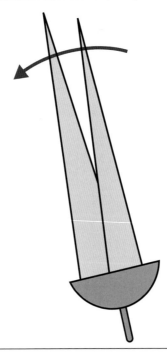

Question: Does it matter how many times I "rock" each vertebra or how quickly?

There is no data to help answer this question. It is important not to overwork any segments of the spine, so rocking each spinous process one to three times seems like an appropriate starting point. The technique should feel soothing to receive, which could equate to about one "rock" per second. This is a good example of where it is useful to receive a technique yourself in order to both appreciate its benefits and experience how it feels to have it applied to your own body.

When you have finished your treatment, it is important to do two things:

- First, reassess your client. Is there an increase in thoracic range of motion? Is there a decrease in symptoms?
- Second, document how many times you "rocked" the spinous processes, and which part of the spine you worked on.

In later treatments, you could experiment with rocking only one side of the spine and retesting to see if this alone has made a positive difference.

Tip 4: Treating Exaggerated Postures of the Thoracic Spine – An Overview

The thoracic spine may be exaggerated in three ways:

- When the natural outward curvature—the kyphosis—of the thoracic spine is exaggerated, a person is said to have a *kyphotic* spine. There are various types of kyphotic spine.
- When the natural kyphosis is diminished, and the back becomes more flat in appearance, this is described as a *flat back*. The term is usually used with reference to a reduced lumbar lordosis.
- Lateral, **C**-shaped or **S**-shaped curvatures combining an exaggeration in the normal kyphosis of the thorax (and an exaggeration of the normal lordosis of the lumbar region) are described as *scoliotic*.

Before reading about some of the treatments, you might employ as a therapist to help a client with an exaggerated kyphosis (Tip 5, pp. 228–229), a flattened thoracic spine (Tip 6, p. 229), or scoliosis (Tip 7, p. 231), it is important to consider three things.

First, ask yourself "What is the rationale for my intervention?"

- It may be to address symptoms you believe are the result of the spinal shape, such as pain, feelings of stiffness, or reduced function.
- It may be purely esthetic, based on the wishes of your client.
- It may be prophylactic, because you believe that with time, the shape of the spine could lead to problems. For example, as

we age, the kyphotic curve becomes more pronounced, the thorax is squashed anteriorly, and our breathing function is impaired due to altered rib mechanics.

Second, although a subject may have a spine with exaggerated curves, this does not necessarily mean that their spine is abnormal. Brunnstrom (1972) notes that the erect, perpendicular posture described by Braune and Fischer (1889) as "Normalstellung" has been incorrectly translated to describe "normal posture," when in fact Braune and Fischer used this term to describe the anatomical relationship of body parts when making measurements. It is interesting that what was an anatomical description of a very erect posture has filtered down through the last century to become a standard for body alignment: the erect posture is now commonly believed to be normal. Therapeutically, postural correction is about alleviating existing symptoms and preventing the likelihood of symptoms occurring in the future without feeling obliged to strive for an esthetic ideal.

Third, the most significant factor in bringing about postural change is what a subject does for themselves on a daily basis. A single, one-off intervention provided by a therapist may be effective but is unlikely to have lasting effect if the change this has facilitated is not maintained by the subject. Chapter 6 provides ideas you can pass on to your clients to help them maintain and improve their posture.

Overview of Treatments

In general terms, treatments for clients with increased kyphosis, flat back, or scoliosis involve the shortening of lengthened muscles and the lengthening of shortened muscles in order to achieve balance in soft tissues and a realignment of joints. This will help both soft tissues and joints to function more optimally. There are many different ways to achieve these, some of which are listed in the following tables.

Examples of ways to shorten lengthened muscles
• Active correction of posture by the client where possible
• Active strengthening using techniques such as: – bodyweight against gravity – exercise bands such as therabands (The Hygenic Corporation) – hand weights – multigym equipment
• Isometric strengthening using techniques such as muscle energy technique, provided that joints are in fairly optimal alignment

Examples of ways to lengthen shortened muscles
• The client adopting resting positions to affect stretch and relaxation of soft tissues
• Passive stretching using techniques such as: – Simple passive stretches – Soft tissue release – Muscle energy technique
• Active stretching of specific body parts, using common stretches or specific techniques such as active soft tissue release
• Correction of posture by the client where this is possible
• Release of trigger points either passively or actively to decrease tone in muscles and facilitate lengthening
• Myofascial release to bring about a relaxation in fascia

Tip 5: **Kyphotic Postures**

A kyphotic posture is one in which the normal kyphotic curve is exaggerated. There are good reasons for wanting to correct excessively kyphotic postures, some of which are the following:

- The imbalance that results can be painful, not only in the upper back, but also in the cervical and lumbar regions, which usually compensate for the kyphosis with an increase in the lordotic curve in these regions.
- The imbalance that results affects the correct functioning of the shoulder because scapulae are usually protracted. Problems such as anterior impingement syndromes in the shoulder and thoracic outlet syndrome are likely to be more common in clients with protracted shoulders. In kyphotic postures, the ability of the trapezius to stabilize the scapulae is compromised.
- The rib cage is depressed, and altered rib function can impair the mechanics of breathing. Abdominal organs are squashed, and this could impair their functioning too.

Muscle Imbalance in Kyphotic Postures	
Shortened muscles	**Lengthened muscles**
Pectoralis major	Rhomboids
Pectoralis minor	Middle fibers of trapezius
Rectus abdominis (upper)	
Posterior neck (where there is associated lordosis in this region)	

Much can be done to correct a kyphotic posture when, for example, it is the result of habitual hunching over a desk, steering wheel, or laptop, or prolonged hunching to perform a hobby. Over the next few pages, you will find information on what you can do for a client with a kyphotic posture and what a client might do for themselves.

The following table provides an overview of treatments for this particular posture. By using the page references in the table, you will be able to locate where particular techniques are described in detail. You will see that most of the suggested techniques for treating people with a kyphotic posture are included in Section 2 of this book as separate tips. This is because they can also be helpful for treating other conditions.

Twelve things you can do for your client with a kyphotic posture	Pages
1. Teach your client the "dart" exercise to strengthen the lower fibers of trapezius and help realign the scapulae	314
2. Teach your client chest stretches	292–295
3. Teach your client thoracic mobility stretches	302–304
4. Teach your client breathing exercises to increase inspiration and improve thoracic mobility	306–309
5. Provide passive chest stretches: – Simple, passive pectoral stretching or – Muscle energy technique stretches to the pectoral muscles (supine or seated) or – Soft tissue release stretches to pectoral muscles (unilaterally and at the sternum)	255–258 259–261 251–253
6. Help relax anterior chest wall muscles using myofascial release	245–246
7. Provide massage with the aim of stretching pectorals	
8. Address trigger points in pectorals	
9. Release tension in upper abdominals	
10. Mobilize the rib cage to encourage improved respiration. This means facilitating correct functioning of the sternocostal and costovertebral joints	269–271
11. Tape the thorax	
12. Refer your client to a fitness professional for strengthening middle and lower fibers of the trapezius and spinal extensors	278–280

Remember that the client is likely to have a lordotic neck and internally rotated shoulders, and these areas also should be addressed. This section of the book focuses on the thorax.

Seven things a client with a kyphotic posture can do for themselves	Pages
1. Strengthen opposing muscle groups with exercises such as the dart. This helps strengthen the lower fibers of trapezius and helps realign the scapulae	314
2. Perform active chest stretches	292–295
3. Perform thoracic mobility stretches	302–304
4. Practice breathing exercises to increase the range of respiration	306–309
5. Alter habits: avoid prolonged kyphotic postures at work or when performing hobbies	310–311
6. Perform exercises to regain correct pelvic alignment: prevent excessive anterior or posterior tilt. The spine is attached to the pelvis by way of the sacrum and the sacroiliac joints, so poor positioning of the pelvis can adversely affect the shape, and therefore the function, of the spine	331
7. Deactivate trigger points in muscles of the anterior thorax	299–301

Tip 6: **Flat Back Postures – in the Thoracic Region**

The normal lumbar lordosis is sometimes flattened, giving rise to the term "flat back." However, you may have come across clients who appear to have a flatter than usual thoracic spine. Such clients may have prominent scapulae and a low body mass index. Such scapulae are sometimes described as "winged" when in fact they simply appear more prominent because the thoracic curve is diminished. These clients often complain of mid-back pain, especially on standing erect or leaning backward. In fact, they may adopt a slight rounding of the shoulders as this alleviates their pain. However, such a posture creates excessive strain on other segments of the spine, such as the C7/T1 region, as posterior neck muscles work to control the forward head position—consequently, therapeutic intervention is often welcomed.

Pain experienced by subjects with thoracic flat back postures may arise because, when standing erect or extending the spine, the spinous processes in this region approximate one another, and soft tissues are squashed.

Five things you can do for a client with a thoracic flat back	Pages
1. Provide general back massage to soothe tensioned muscles, including **S** bends to release tension	234–235
2. Rock spinous processes to decrease muscle spasm and alleviate pain	223–225
3. Address trigger points in erector spinae, rhomboids, or middle fibers of trapezius	
4. Passively stretch the latissimus dorsi	
5. Perform longitudinal stretches to ease tension in soft tissues of the posterior spine	232–233

Three things a client with a thoracic flat back can do for themselves	Pages
1. Avoid extending their spine	
2. Active stretches for erector spinae, rhomboids, and middle fibers of trapezius	296–298
3. Self-trigger of the posterior thorax	299–301

Tip 7: **Scoliotic Postures**

Whether a person has a **C**-shaped or an **S**-shaped scoliosis, there are physiological (as opposed to esthetic) reasons for correction of an excessively scoliotic posture. In such postures:

- Internal organs become displaced and their function may be compromised.
- Spinal nerves may be pinched where they exit the vertebral canal.
- The spine's ability to support body-weight is reduced by lateral curvature.

Hartvig Nissen was a firm believer in the use of exercise to help correct scoliosis, and in his book, *Practical Massage and Corrective Exercises* (1905), he provides examples of the assessments he made of children with scoliosis "before" and "after" his treatment using specific sets of exercises. The black and white photographs of Nissen demonstrating his "corrective" exercises, with his beard and bow tie and high-waisted trousers, are amusing to the modern eye. But Nissen was a massage therapist also and is to be applauded for being brave enough to publish what he claimed were his findings based on 30 years' experience. Solberg (2008) notes that in 1941 the American Orthopaedic Association concluded exercises should not be used in the treatment of scoliosis, on the basis that studies showed exercise failed to halt the progress of the condition. However, Solberg does a good job in clarifying some of the research on this topic. She notes that when methodological flaws were eliminated and the studies were repeated, exercise *did* have a positive effect on scoliotic postures, arguing (on p. 107) that, "Therapeutic exercise may actually produce improvement in the scoliosis and engender significant change both in body posture and in general functioning of the spinal column." Perhaps Nissen was right all along.

It is hardly surprising that there are conflicting views regarding the use of exercise to correct scoliosis. Flaws in exercise programs, whether for the treatment of scoliosis or other conditions, are common. For example, incorrect exercises may be prescribed in the first place; the exercise may be correct, but the intensity or duration wrong; the subject may perform the prescribed exercises incorrectly or they may forget to perform them at all. Notably, as a client's condition changes, exercises need to be modified. Therapeutic exercises for scoliosis are not included in this section because there is more than one type of scoliosis, and "corrective" exercise programs need to be individually tailored and delivered by professionals specialized in this field.

Things you can do for a client with scoliotic posture		
• Massage and stretching of shortened tissues		

• Referral to a specialist practitioner for corrective exercise	For more information, contact:
	The British Orthopaedic Association,
	    http://www.boa.ac.uk/
	The American Orthopaedic Association,
	    http://www.aoassn.org/	

Things the client can do for themselves		**Page**
• Practice corrective postures		313

Tip 8: Longitudinal Stretches for Flat Back

When treating a client with a flattened thoracic curve, the erector spinae muscles are shortened compared to those of a client with a normal thoracic curve. The purpose of this technique is to stretch out these shortened tissues, focusing on the midline region and the spinalis thoracic muscle.

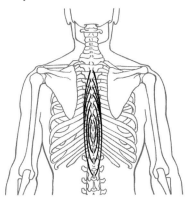

STEP 2 Place one hand on the base of the skull and one on the sacrum and apply gentle traction. Your aim is to gently traction the skin, fascia, and maybe even underlying muscle. Patience is required as you settle into a comfortable hand position and wait for tissues to yield.

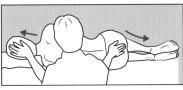

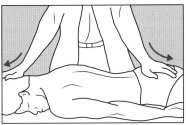

STEP 1 Select the side-lying or the prone position. If using the side-lying position, your client needs to flex at both the hips and knees by about 90 degrees; if using the prone position, they need to tuck their chin toward their chest.

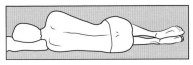

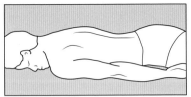

Question: Is this the same as the dural tube stretch used in myofascial release?

No. Although the subtle stretch described here utilizes the same position as a myofascial release dural tube stretch, they are not the same. The aim here is not to release the dural tube but the spinal extensor muscles in the midline region.

Alternatives are to get the client to turn their head to one side (a), to apply a diagonal stretch (b), or to apply the stretch with your arms crossed (c).

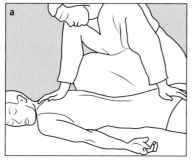

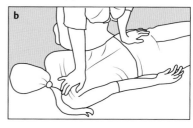

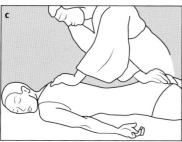

TIP: Lower your treatment couch for this technique or practice it on the floor. Experiment to see which position is most comfortable to receive.

Tip 9: "S" Strokes

This soft tissue technique is also particularly useful for clients with tension in the midline, such as clients with a flattened kyphotic curve. It is soothing to receive and may therefore be incorporated into a general back massage routine.

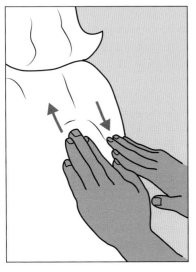
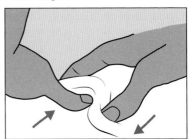

With your client prone, and without using any medium (such as wax or oil), gently stretch the tissues on either side of the spinous processes by using your fingers to create **S** shapes as you push the skin upward (cephalad) on one side and downward (caudal) on the other.

Question: Do I need to start at the top of the thoracic spine and work down, or at the bottom of the thorax and work up?

It does not matter where you start.

Question: Do I alternate the **S** shapes so that I am pushing up on one side of the spine and then pushing down on that same side?

You could perform the same stroke from one end of the spine to the other and then reverse. So, for example, if you start by pushing up on the left of the spine and down on the right from the lumbar spine to the neck (a), when you reach the neck, change your position and push the tissues down on the left and up on the right (b), as shown in the figures below.

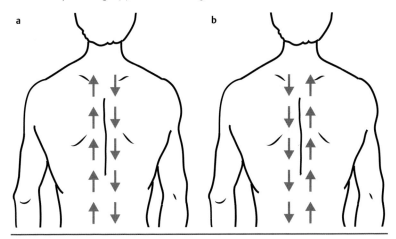

Tip 10: Addressing Tension in Erector Spinae

Erector spinae are spinal extensors as you know. They are active all of the time we are sitting, standing, walking, or engaged in sport or physical activity. Observing that a client has enlarged erector spinae muscles does not mean that there is anything wrong with these muscles. We would not attempt to dampen down the tone in the muscles of a client who had, for example, nicely developed biceps, would we? So it is strange that many therapists feel they need to reduce the size of a client's erector spinae muscles by "working" them, rubbing the muscles, "twanging" them like guitar strings, or circling them with friction type movements in an attempt to flatten them out.

However, it *would* be appropriate to try and reduce tone in erector spinae where the increase in tone is the source of pain. Often this occurs where tone is localized to a short segment of muscle. It would also be appropriate to try and decrease tone where you believe hypertrophy of the muscle is contributing to muscle imbalance.

As with all manual techniques, if you don't find the routine here helpful, then simply don't use it; if you like it, practice with it for several sessions, with several different clients or work with a colleague and receive the routine yourself.

Suggested Routine to Decrease Tone in Erector Spinae

With your client in the prone position, covered with a towel, you can perform the following routine:

- **Work through the towel:**
  1. *Rocking* With a towel draped over your client, without touching the back itself, place your hands on the sides of the thorax, arms, hips, or legs and gently rock your subject for about a minute, working down one side of the body and up the other side. Use gentle, rhythmic rocking of low amplitude. For more information on rocking, see Tip 22: Rocking (p. 281).

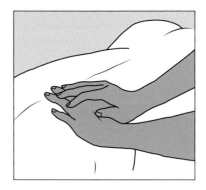

2. *Stillness* Place your hands on the thorax and wait. Have you noticed how, when you are in an environment that is very still, such as a monastery, empty beach, or in the countryside, the stillness of the moment is transmitted to you? After gentle rocking, allow your client to sense the stillness within you.

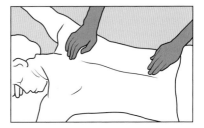

TIP: It is useful to practice visualizing your own favorite still place as you perform this technique.

---

3. *Compression* Gently lean onto your client, transferring your weight through either your hands (a), reinforced palms (b), or forearm (c), and then lean off your client. Repeat this several times, without moving your hands. This gentle compression–release–compression–release is calming. Move your hands (or forearms) to two different positions on the back and repeat the technique.

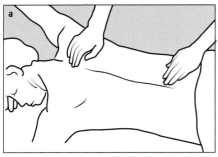

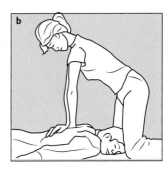

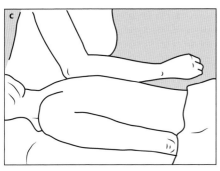

- **Remove the towel and apply a massage medium such as oil or wax:**

  4. *Massage* Using effleurage only, massage the back. As you massage, notice which parts of the erector spinae seem to have an increase in tone or which parts the client reports are uncomfortable. Continue with this routine.

- **Replace the towel:**

  Now that a massage medium is on the skin, it will "grip" the towel and provide a greater degree of traction. This will enable you to compress and stretch tissues using less pressure than usual.

TIP: Compare how it feels both to give and to receive the next technique first *through a towel* after oil has been applied, and then *on skin* after oil has been applied.

---

5. *Transverse stretch* Standing to one side of the client, locate the spinous processes. Working through the towel, using the thenar eminence of your palm, gently "lock" the soft tissues on the opposite side of the spine to which you are standing and push the erector spinae away from the spine.

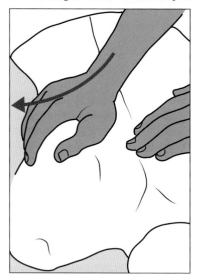 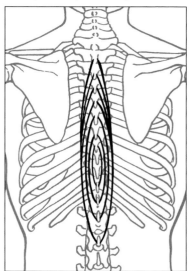

It doesn't matter where you start and you can overlap each stretch a little. Repeat two or three times on each side of the spine. It doesn't matter whether you work up and down on one side of the spine before moving to the other side or feel comfortable working alternate sides of the spine, working up one side and down the other. Avoid "twanging" the erector spinae. Well-meaning therapists sometimes overwork the muscle and the result is an increase rather than a decrease in tone. This may be because the "twanging" movement has a stimulatory rather than an inhibitory effect.

6. *Massage* Reapply your massage medium and massage the back for a few minutes. Note whether there feels to be a decrease in tone anywhere.

7. *Longitudinal "stripping"* Stand to one side of your client and, starting at the lumbar region or low thorax, gently run a reinforced thumb or fingers up the erector spinae, going slower than you would normally.

When you reach a section of increased tone, simply pause. Sometimes the tone will decrease as a trigger spot gets released. If not, reduce your pressure, move over the spot, and continue in this slow manner. You could use your elbow but remember to guide it as you move slowly up the erector spinae muscles.

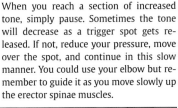

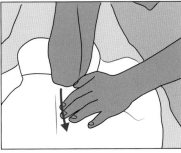

8. *Massage* Finish with effleurage, and reevaluate your client's symptoms.

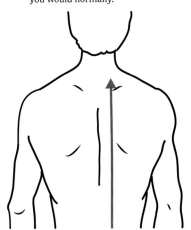

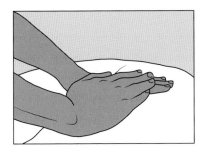

TIP: It is helpful to practice this sequence with two other people: one person to receive the treatment, one person to provide the treatment, and a third person to read out each technique.

Tip 11: Overcoming Spasm in Thoracic Muscles

Have you ever experienced muscle spasm? In the thoracic region this is sometimes felt:

- In the upper part of rectus abdominis where it attaches to the costal cartilages near the midline. If you have ever been hunched, your spine flexed, you may have experienced spasm here.
- In an intercostal where it is often described as a "stitch" on the lateral side of the thorax.
- In the obliques, where they attach laterally at the costal cartilages.
- In the thoracic erector spinae. You may have treated a client who tells you that their back goes into "spasm" (although this is often in the lumbar, rather than thoracic region).

With time, the spasm subsides, but it can be excruciatingly painful. This tip describes different ways of overcoming sudden muscle spasm in the thorax. The techniques described here may also be used to overcome an increase in tone in localized segments of the thoracic muscles. While a spasm is an involuntary, painful, and temporary contraction of muscle, perhaps lasting a minute or two, a localized increase in tone can occur for longer durations, and is not necessarily painful. A localized increase in tone may develop where muscles are guarding underlying structures that may not be functioning correctly. In the lumbar region, a common example is where the client suffers a disk herniation, and there is an immediate spasming of surrounding muscles. The spasm is painful and pain may subside with time, but the increase in tone remains. Similarly, following a blow to the thigh there may be damage to muscle tissue leading to an increase in tone that is palpable superior and inferior to this localized spot of trauma. Such an increase in tone is not necessarily painful.

There are five ways to overcome spasm in the thoracic region, which are as follows:

1. Stretch the muscle in question
2. Apply static pressure
3. Apply static pressure *and* stretch
4. Isometric contraction or concentric contraction of the opposing muscle group
5. Apply positional release technique

Let us look at each of the treatments in turn.

Question: What causes muscles to spasm?

It is not clear what causes a muscle to spasm. Some of the contributing factors include the following:

- Retaining a shortened position. Muscles tend to cramp more frequently when they have been kept either actively or passively shortened.
- Dehydration. Cramps are more likely to occur when a subject is dehydrated.
- Electrolyte imbalance. Muscles require not only water, but also glucose, sodium, potassium, calcium, and magnesium. Inadequate supplies of these nutrients could contribute to cramp.
- Fatigue. Cramps are more likely to occur when a muscle is overused and tired. The muscle's energy stores are depleted and it becomes hyperexcitable.
- Repetitive motion of the same muscle.
- Abnormalities in the size of blood vessels. While this may affect muscles in the legs, it is unlikely to affect muscles of the back.
- Some illnesses (e.g., anemia, diabetes, multiple sclerosis).
- Hormonal abnormalities.
- Stress and anxiety.
- Caffeine.
- Some medicines.

1. *Stretch the muscle in question:* The table on the following pages provides some ideas as to how to stretch out a spasming muscle in the thorax, focusing on those muscles in which cramps commonly occur in this part of the body:
   - The upper part of rectus abdominis or an anterior intercostal muscle.
   - An oblique or lateral intercostal muscle.
   - Muscles of thoracic extension.

Suggestions have been made for stretches that could be performed sitting, standing, lying, and, in some cases, in alternative positions because the client may be at work, at home, or outdoors when they experience a cramp and so it is useful for them to know alternative positions in which to stretch.

If you have a client prone to spasm in the thoracic region, help educate them as to how they could use these stretches to treat a spasm.

	Sitting	Standing
Upper part of rectus abdominis or an anterior intercostal		
Oblique or lateral intercostal (These examples show the stretch to overcome spasm on the left side)		
Thoracic extensor		

	On floor	Other
Upper part of rectus abdominis or an anterior intercostal		
Oblique or lateral intercostal (These examples show the stretch to overcome spasm on the left side)		
Thoracic extensor		

Question: Why are there no passive stretches illustrated?

This is for three reasons.

First, stretching the muscles listed requires the spine to be extended (to stretch abdominals), rotated and extended (to stretch obliques), or flexed (to stretch extensors). Passively stretching the spine in extension, rotation, and flexion needs to be done with great care and may not have been included in the training general massage therapists have received. As this book is designed primarily with students and newly qualified therapists in mind, passive spine stretches have been omitted.

Second, spasm in thoracic muscles is less likely to occur during a massage treatment than in muscles of the hamstrings, calves, and feet, so the therapist is not necessarily going to be present to provide the stretch when the spasm occurs.

Third, there are alternative techniques that can be provided by a therapist (see pp. 243–244), which are arguably better to alleviate spasm.

2. *Static pressure*: This simply involves applying pressure directly to the spasming muscle, over the site of pain. If you have ever experienced cramp, you will know that we instinctively press the painful spot to try and alleviate the pain.

If a client experiences cramp while you are treating them, one of the best ways to alleviate it is to apply static pressure at a 90-degree angle to the tissue, using fingertip or thumb pressure.

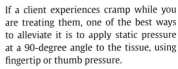

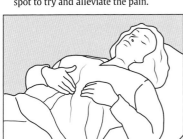

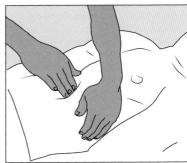

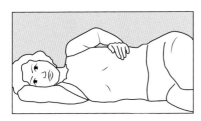

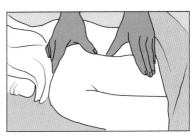

3. *Static pressure and stretch*: By combining a static pressure with stretch, you are performing a pin-and-lock or soft tissue release (STR) technique and this too is effective at helping to overcome cramp. The client may perform this themselves. For example, for abdominal cramp they would apply pressure to the area of pain (usually beneath the anterior ribs) and lean backward, arching their back, stretching the abdominals as they continue to apply pressure.

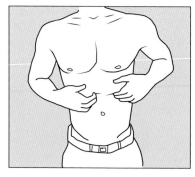

For cramp in an intercostal, they need to apply pressure and lean *away* from the side of pain.

4. *Isometric contraction or concentric contraction of the opposing muscle group*: Contracting the antagonist of the spasming muscle is yet another way to reduce the pain of cramp. For example, if spasm occurs in the superior portion of the rectus abdominis muscle, the client needs to contract the antagonists, which in this case are the erector spinae group. This may mean instructing the client to press their back into a wall or the back of a chair. Actively engaging the antagonist reduces tone (and cramp) in the agonist (the cramping muscle).

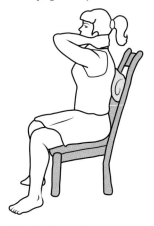

5. *Positional release technique*: This is the opposite of the STR pin-and-lock technique. Instead of trying to stretch out the cramping muscle, encourage your client to lean into it, shortening the muscle until they find a position of ease. If the cramp occurred in the abdominals, the client would flex at the waist; if it occurred in the side of the thorax, they would flex *to the side of the pain*.

Question: What else can I do to help my client avoid cramp in their thoracic muscles?

There are two things you can advise the client to do.

First, that they avoid postures likely to trigger spasm, especially following exercise. For example, if the abdominal cramp occurs when removing shoes following a run, suggest that your client stretches their abdominals or waits for 10 minutes after their run before removing their shoes. If a client's cramp occurs to one side of their thorax, in the intercostals or obliques, help them ensure that they are not rotated to one side for long periods as might happen during work or a hobby.

Second, suggest that your client ensure they are properly hydrated and that they address any nutritional deficiencies they might have. They should take medical advice if medication could be a contributing factor.

Tip 12: **Myofascial Release Techniques to the Thorax**

In a book of this size, it is only possible to touch briefly on different techniques but, in order to illustrate the wide variety of treatment approaches that you could explore, a small selection of myofascial release (MFR) techniques has been included.

Superficial Release

If you have used the assessment described in Chapter 4, Tip 25: Assessment of Superficial Fascia (p. 213) and found superficial restrictions between the skin and underlying fascia, you could use a release technique from Manheim and Lavett (1989). They describe how superficial restrictions can be released by making J-shaped strokes across the restriction, using one hand to fix and stretch the tissues above the restriction in an upward direction, as you "draw" short Js on the patient's skin, progressively moving across the restricted area. Assess the tissues again using fingertips or your palm as in Tip 25 and repeat with J strokes until no more restrictions can be felt.

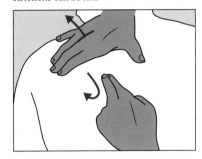

Cross-Hand Techniques

A popular approach is to apply a cross-hand technique over whichever section of the thorax you are working. This could be the ribs in side lying, the back in prone, or the chest in supine. In all cases, the steps are simple.

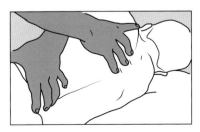

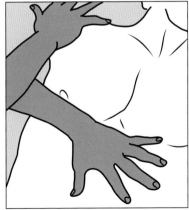

STEP 1 Stand wherever you are most comfortable, your hands crossed, without using any massage medium. Allow your hands to rest on the skin and focus your attention here as they begin to "sink" into the tissues as the tissues soften.

STEP 2 As you wait, avoid pressing into the tissues, but be patient and follow any movement that you feel beneath your hands, maintaining contact with the skin.

Compressive Technique

This could be applied supine or seated. For example, while sitting at the side of the couch, place one hand on the sternum and the other on the posterior thorax, with both palms touching the skin. Wait for your client to relax and to acclimate to your touch. Once you feel tissues soften and you begin to sink into them, apply subtle pressure with your uppermost hand. Sit in this posture and note any twitches or changes that occur in your client.

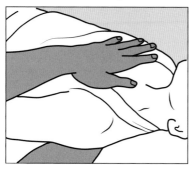

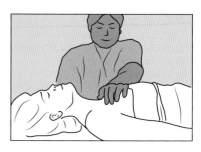

For Lateral Bends in the Spine

You could work specifically at various segments of the spine, using your fingertips to apply gentle pressure to the soft tissues. Earls and Myers (2010) describe how to use MFR to help normalize the erector tissues either side of a spinal bend. For example, working with a client with a curve to the right, the tissues on the convex side are farther away from the spine, so you would encourage these to glide medially, whereas the tissues on the convex side of the spine are closer to the spine, so you would encourage these to glide laterally, thus helping to bring about balance in the position of tissues. The technique is described with the client sitting, leaning away from the side on which you are working as you engage the tissues. For a full explanation of this and other thoracic techniques, please refer to their text.

Example of Treatment to Address Spinal Curvature to the Right		
	Position of tissues	**Treatment aim**
Convex side of the curve	Medial erector spinae muscles are farther away from spine	Glide tissues medially
Concave side of the curve	Medial erector spinae muscles are closer to spine	Glide tissues laterally

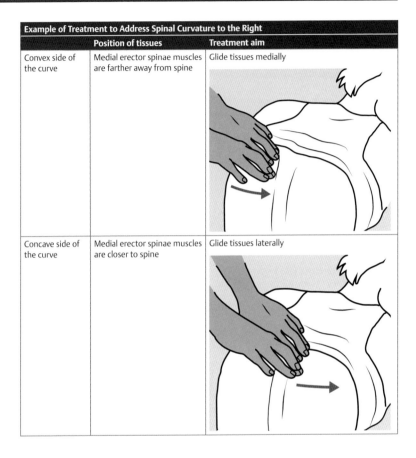

Addressing Thoracic Rotations

Another MFR technique is described by Duncan (2012) to address rotations in the thorax.

Note that in this technique there is no skin drag or traction; this is a mechanical movement.

STEP 1 Standing to one side of the treatment couch, place your hands just below the manubrium and on the lower ribs. As with other MFR techniques, allow your hands to feel into the tissues, sink into them as you apply subtle pressure.

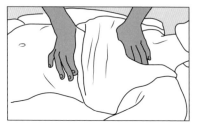

STEP 2 Gently roll the thorax away from you and then toward you.

Decide which direction feels most restricted. If the restriction is as you roll away from you, remain where you are standing. If you sense that the restriction was as you rolled toward you, move to the other side of the couch and begin your treatment there as it is easier to roll a client away from you than toward you when performing step 4.

STEP 3 Once you have decided where to stand, begin again, taking your time to sink into the tissues and then roll the rib cage first to where it feels *easiest*, which should be *toward you* if you are standing in the correct position.

STEP 4 Now start to work on the area of *restriction*. Remaining where you are, roll the rib cage away from you until you sense a barrier. Wait there until you feel up to three "releases" as you remain in the same position.

The following table provides an overview to help you decide where to stand and in which direction to roll your client.

Restriction felt as you roll your client to *their* left	
Stand on right of your client	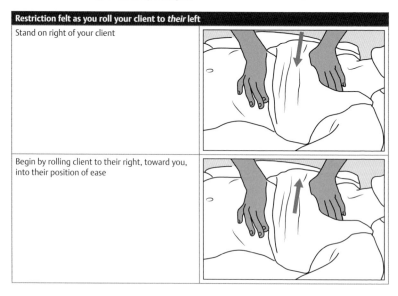
Begin by rolling client to their right, toward you, into their position of ease	

Roll client to their left, away from you, into the restriction. Wait for 2–3 "releases"	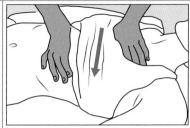

Restriction felt as you roll your client to *their* right

Stand on left of your client	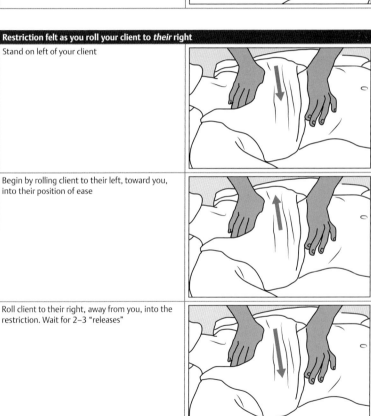
Begin by rolling client to their left, toward you, into their position of ease	
Roll client to their right, away from you, into the restriction. Wait for 2–3 "releases"	

Tip 13: **Soft Tissue Release to the Thorax**

Soft tissue release (STR) is a technique that may be used to gently stretch soft tissues by first forming a "lock" and then, while maintaining this lock, moving the body actively or passively to bring about a stretch.

Applying Soft Tissue Release to Rhomboids

STEP 1 Position your client so that they are at an angle on the treatment couch. Passively extend the arm.

STEP 2 Apply gentle pressure to the tissues, taking up some slack in the tissue by pushing it from the medial border of the scapula toward the spine.

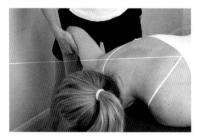

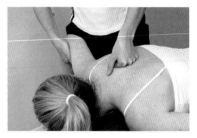

TIP: Note that the scapula needs to be able to protract, and to do this, the arm must be able to flex. The only way to do this in the prone position is for your client to be positioned with their shoulder to the side of the couch. You can see that while the advantage of this technique is that it enables you to apply STR in the prone position, the disadvantage is that in order to apply the technique to the opposite side of the body you need to reposition your client, which disrupts the normal flow of a treatment.

STEP 3 Maintaining your lock, lower the arm. Notice the awkwardness of the therapist's position as she does this. An alternative is to lock the tissues using your fingers, fist, or reinforced thumbs and then to let the client lower their own arm.

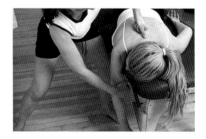

The key to this technique working successfully is for you to maintain traction in the soft tissues as you glide these toward the spine, rather than pressing down through them and onto the ribs.

Question: Is it possible to apply STR to rhomboids with a client seated?

Yes. Like when treating in the prone position, you passively retract the scapula, and to do this with a seated client, you need to support the whole of their arm and gently draw the shoulder into extension, retracting the scapula. You then take up some slack in the skin of the scapula closest to you, drawing it from the medial border toward the spine, and keep it fixed. In this position, you then ask the client to bring their arm forward again as if to give themselves a hug. The difficulty with applying STR with the client seated is that you have less leverage and tend to push the client forward as you fix the soft tissues in order to get a lock.

Applying Soft Tissue Release to Pectorals

STEP 1 With your client supine, select a spot over the pectoral muscles and lock it gently, using fingertips or a soft fist once you have passively shortened the muscle. Gently push the tissues away from you, taking up some of the slack.

STEP 2 Ask your client to gently take back their arm as shown, stopping if the stretch is too severe.

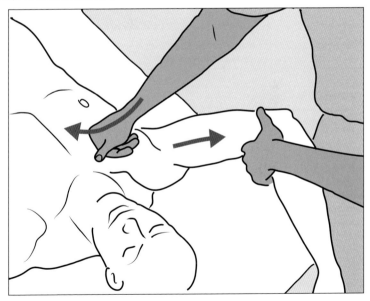

Question: Does my client need to keep their elbow extended during shoulder movement?

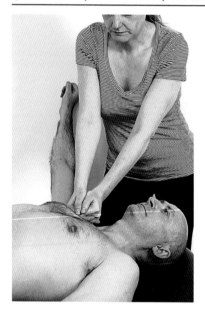 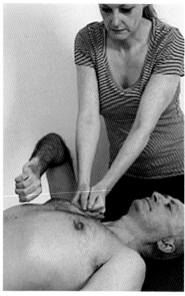

No. The stretch is sometimes felt more greatly when the elbow is extended because it can be felt in the tissues of the anterior arm, elbow, and forearm.

TIP: You need to play around with where you stand because you need to provide space for your client to move their arm. Sometimes it works better to stand at the head of the couch rather than to the side.

Bilateral Soft Tissue Release to Medial Pectoral Tissues

This is a method of gently stretching soft tissues bilaterally, working in the intercostal spaces, from the superior to the inferior portion of the sternum. Even though it may be performed through a T-shirt or towel, you may feel that it is not appropriate for all clients.

STEP 1 With your client in the supine position, stand at the head of the couch and ask them to flex their shoulders so that they have both arms out in front of them, flexed at the shoulder by about 90 degrees. Gently palpate the sternum and then discover the intercostal spaces. It is into these spaces that you are going to place a fingertip on each side.

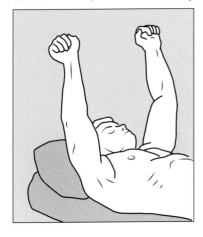

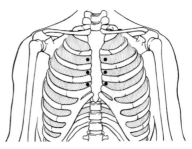

STEP 2 With a fingertip in the intercostal space on each side of the sternum, gently lock the tissue of the sternum, gliding it toward the sternum itself, and ask your client to abduct their arms.

Question: How far down the sternum do I work?

This depends on how comfortable your client feels receiving this technique and how far you can reach down the sternum without discomfort to yourself. As very little pressure is required and the technique does not take more than about a minute to apply, you are likely to be able to work superiorly to inferiorly quite easily. However, avoid pressing the xiphoid process itself at the very end of the sternum.

Soft Tissue Release to Posterior Tissues

This is a good example of where the line between STR and MFR is blurred with regard to the application of the technique. If you are a sports massage therapist, you may know this as a soft tissue technique and may use it both with and without oil; if you use predominantly MFR you may know this as MFR and may be used to using it on dry skin.

STEP 1 With your client seated on a stool or bench, have them sit upright and gently place the back of your fists on the upper thorax to either side of the spine. The technique works well if you can apply your pressure at a 90-degree angle to the body.

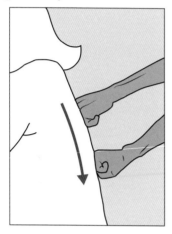

STEP 2 Beginning at the upper thorax, ask your client to curl their body slowly forward one vertebra at a time, flexing their spine. As they do this, glide slowly down their back until you reach the sacrum.

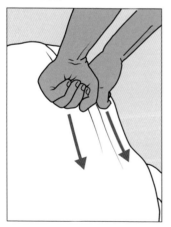

An alternative is to work in a localized spot. To save your thumbs and fingers, lock the tissues with gentle pressure using your elbows, making sure not to press on the spinous processes of the vertebrae. Once you have locked the tissues, ask your client to flex their neck. You will notice that using this method you cannot work as far down the spine as when you use your fists.

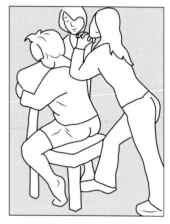

Notice that if you press too hard, you risk pushing your client forward and so forcing them to press back against you. You do not need to apply a lot of pressure for this technique to be effective (see Johnson 2009).

Tip 14: Passive Pectoral Stretches

There are many ways to passively stretch thoracic muscles. The position you choose depends on your client's preferences and where you are treating them. It is important to remember that whichever position you choose, the more relaxed your client is, the more effective will be your stretch.

Two of the most common mistakes therapists make when stretching pectoral muscles are the following:

• *Stretching too quickly*: If you move the shoulder joint too quickly into a position of tension and apply too much force, the result is that the client contracts their muscles in a bid to protect their shoulder. Remember, if a client has been working with their arms in front of themselves, hunched at a desk or engaged in sport or strenuous physical activity involving the upper body, their muscles may be shortened and tense. It is important to *slowly* take the upper limb into a stretch position, find the barrier point gradually and sensitively, and apply gentle force.

• *Not holding the stretch long enough*: Finding a barrier point and waiting a few seconds is not a passive stretch. You need to find the point, hold the stretch, and *feel* the tissues release. This takes longer for some clients than others and clients used to receiving passive stretches will relax more quickly than those who are not used to receiving them. So give yourself and your client time to experience the stretch.

Passive Pectoral Stretches in the Supine Position

One of the simplest stretches, with your client resting in the supine position, is to gently abduct your client's arm and apply gently pressure.

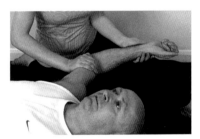

This is only effective if your client has particularly short pectorals: if they can perform active chest stretches such as those shown in Chapter 6, Tip 1 (pp. 292–295) without feeling much of a stretch, then this position is unlikely to be effective.

An alternative is for your client to position their hand behind their head. In this position, the stretch is felt much more in the armpit and lower fibers of pectoralis major.

This stretch is good when you want to stretch only one side of a pectoral at a time or perhaps when a client has an upper limb problem and stretching the affected side is contraindicated.

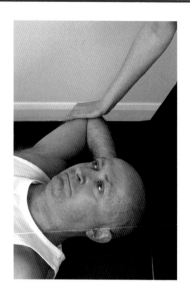

Passive Pectoral Stretches in the Sitting Position

When your client can receive a full pectoral stretch, this could be applied in the sitting position. Experiment with different handholds and positions (shown in the illustration below), such as back to front with hands over the elbows (a), back to front with hands beneath the elbows (b), or back to back (c and d).

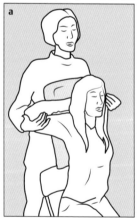

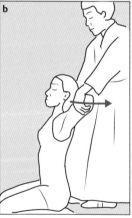

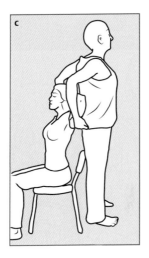
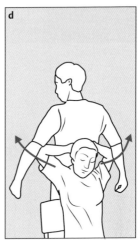

TIP: You are aiming to "open" the chest, not to extend the spine. Some spinal extension is inevitable, but it is a mistake to try and apply a passive chest stretch while at the same time extending the client's spine, whether this is intentional or not. For most clients a combined pectoral-and-extension stretch is too severe.

Experiment also with using seats of different heights, such as chairs and stools, or with the client sitting or kneeling on the floor.

Use the following table as a simple guide to help you practice with a partner using three different handholds in two different sitting positions:

  A On a regular chair.

  B On a low chair or stool.

You could use the cells beneath the illustrations simply to add a tick to show that you have practiced the stretch or to scribble a few notes about how this stretch felt to apply.

Remember also to receive the stretch yourself and notice how you feel. Do both you and your practice partner enjoy applying the technique in the same manner? In which treatment position and with which handholds did you feel most comfortable to receive the technique? Do you and your partner agree or differ?

Back to front with therapist's hands over top of client's elbows	Back to front with therapist's hands beneath client's elbows	Back to back
A		
B		

Tip 15: Muscle Energy Technique for Pectorals

Muscle energy technique (MET) can be used as a means of strengthening the pectorals or as a stretch. When used for strengthening, MET is particularly useful following injury and may be used with very low levels of isometric contraction to facilitate healing. However, injury to pectoral muscles is less common than to other parts of the body and so the MET described here is that for stretching. Many clients present with "tight" pectorals, and helping to stretch these tissues is beneficial because it helps correct muscle imbalance and reduces the likelihood of anterior shoulder impingements.

Remember that if you are applying the stretch to one side only, you need to position your client so that they can extend their shoulder. This means positioning them so that they rest at an angle on the treatment couch, perhaps horizontally, so that the side being treated is closest to the edge of the couch. Whether you choose to apply this stretch to one side of the body at a time or to the whole of the chest at the same time, the principles are the same.

Applying MET unilaterally is useful when the client cannot receive MET to the other side of the chest, perhaps due to a shoulder injury. It is also recommended when treating clients who are particularly strong, as in this position you have considerable leverage as a therapist.

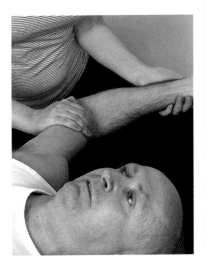

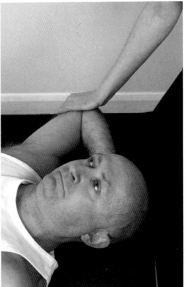

Where a client can receive MET bilaterally, this saves time. Standing back to back is particularly useful when stretching clients who have strong pectorals because this position affords you considerable leverage. When treating such clients, consider comparing this position with that of the unilateral position and see which you and your client prefer.

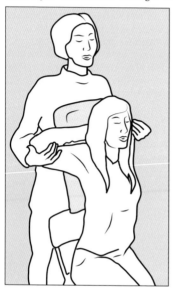

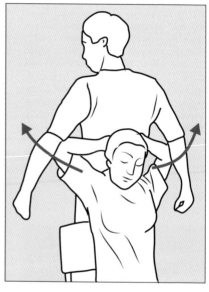

Remember that you are attempting to "open" the chest by stretching the pectorals, not extending the spine. Placing a bolster or pillow lengthwise, behind the client, between their back and the chair, is useful in overcoming this.

STEP 1 With the client in a comfortable position, either supine or seated, gently take their arm to the barrier point. This is where the client feels the tension in their muscle increasing ahead of the muscle being stretched. This is your start position.

STEP 2 Ask your client to contract their muscle, using about 10% of their force. How they do this will depend on the position in which you are treating them. If seated, ask them to try to bring their elbows forward, closing them; if they are

supine, they should try to bring the elbow that is off the couch back to the midline, as if using a pectoral machine in a gym.

For this stretch, you resist the client, and maintain their position even though they are contracting slightly. It is important to remember that you resist the client and that the client should never be trying to resist you, to overcome your force. It is your client who determines how strong "10%" of their force is, not you. A common mistake made by practitioners is to start pulling (if the client is seated) or pushing (if the client is supine) the arms back, overcoming the client's force and causing the client to contract more strongly than they would otherwise do. This is counterproductive as it fatigues the client and prevents the low levels of contraction necessary when using MET techniques.

STEP 3 After about 10 to 12 seconds of contractions, ask your client to relax, then gently stretch their muscle. Hold them in this new position, making sure that you only stretch to the point they are comfortable. Repeat 1–2 more times.

TIP: Some clients experience tingling in their arms when MET is applied bilaterally in sitting. This is simply the result of temporary compression of neurovascular structures and disappears when the client shakes out their arms following the stretch.

Question: Are there any contraindications to MET to the pectorals?

MET is not appropriate for clients with acute neck or shoulder injuries, nor for clients with greatly reduced range of movement in their shoulder. MET to the pectorals while standing back to back is not possible for clients with adhesive capsulitis (although it is greatly beneficial in other treatment positions). MET for the purposes of stretching is not appropriate for clients with shoulder dislocation or subluxation or for clients who are hypermobile. These clients would benefit more from MET to strengthen muscles of the shoulder joint rather than stretching of the pectorals.

Tip 16: **Working the Medial Border**

Many of us use subscapular techniques as part of our treatment for the upper back. If you are reading this as a student of osteopathy or physiotherapy, you will learn more about joint mobilization techniques. It is nevertheless useful to know how to work the tissues around the medial border of the scapula because it is important to release soft tissue restrictions before attempting joint mobilizations of the thoracic spine. By accessing the medial border of the scapula, it is possible to focus a treatment through the middle fibers of trapezius into rhomboid muscles.

There are many different ways to access this border. This tip is included in the hope that it will give you some ideas as to how you might modify your own treatments if you have been struggling with this region of the back.

Taking the Client's Arm behind Them

Many therapists learn to take the client's arm gently behind the client's back in order to make the medial border more prominent. In many cases, this does make the border more prominent.

However, unless the arm and shoulder are properly supported, the client is likely to contract the rhomboid muscles, not intentionally, but in an attempt to stabilize their arm. The result is that therapists often identify the rhomboids as being tight, and assume this is a muscular defect, when in fact it could be because the client is being forced to produce an isometric contraction of these muscles due to the treatment position.

sometimes prevent their arm from slipping off their back, down onto the treatment couch, something that frequently happens if you are using oil and are not holding their arm or hand.

Some therapists hold the client's arm as they work the medial border, but this may not offer enough support.

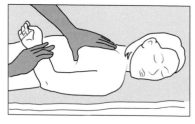

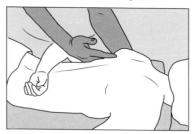

By placing a sponge or small pillow between yourself and your client, you can

To overcome this problem, simply add a small pillow, bolster, or rolled-up towel *beneath the anterior part of the shoulder* when treating your client in the prone position with their arm behind them. In this way, the shoulder is prevented from falling forward onto the couch as it normally would in the prone position; the upper and middle fibers are restored to a more neutral position, decreasing tension on these structures.

Question: Why can't I just hold the client's arm in the extended position as I massage around the medial border?

There are two reasons why this is less preferable than supporting the shoulder with a sponge or towel. The first is that you compromise your own posture when trying to support the client's arm with one of your arms while massaging the medial border with your other arm because it requires you to lean toward the client and twist at the waist. The second reason is that many therapists think they are supporting the client's arm but in fact they are not; the elbow particularly is left unsupported. You can practice for yourself to see in which position the rhomboids feel most tense and decide for yourself which position you prefer.

Techniques in Prone

Once you have decided you wish to access the medial border with your client in the prone position, you have a range of techniques you could use. These include applying pressure with fingers (a), thumbs (b), forearm (c), the side of your hand (d), or the web of your hand (e). Each of these has advantages and disadvantages.

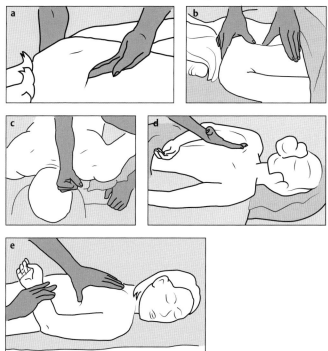

Working in the Side-Lying Position

This could be used as part of your treatment, hooking your fingers under the medial border to give a gentle passive stretch to rhomboids.

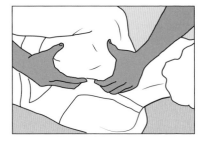

TIP: If you use this, you need to get as close as possible to your client, and it is a good idea to place a pillow between you both for comfort because there is a tendency to ease the client toward you as you stretch the tissues. Be cautious with this stretch because the client's bodyweight is the weight against which the rhomboids are tractioned, so always work slowly and with care.

Sometimes in the side-lying position, you can gently palpate the border, and this works especially well if you let the client's arm rest on their side or slightly behind them, passively shortening the scapular retractors.

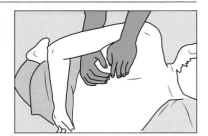

Question: What can I do if I can't get hold of the scapula in this way?

You can work through a towel, something that is especially helpful if you have been using oil or wax and the skin is slippery. Working through a towel will enable you to "grip" the tissues. Remember, however, that not all techniques are appropriate for all clients, and there are plenty of others you could try if this one feels awkward.

In the Sitting Position

Pressing up and under the scapula is a useful technique, but it is difficult to achieve in some clients and when working with female clients, may cause problems with towel draping.

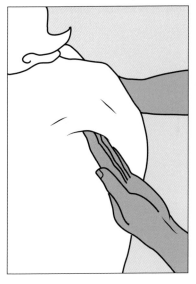 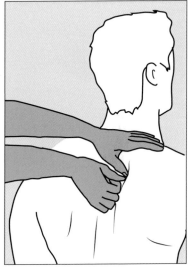

With your client sitting, there is a tendency to push them forward whenever you apply anything but the lightest pressure to the back, so they are never fully relaxed. A way to overcome this is to place one hand on the front of their shoulder to help stabilize them.

TRICK: Notice that if you gently palpate tender spots along the medial border, you can request that your subject move their shoulder *onto* your thumbs. To do this, they push their shoulder blade backward, onto you. Alternatively, without oil, you can fix a spot and ask your subject to elevate, depress, or protract their shoulder as you find a way to stretch their soft tissues in a very localized spot.

Question: My client complains that it is uncomfortable when I take their arm behind them. What should I do?

You do not need to incorporate every technique you have learned into every treatment. Ask yourself why you are attempting this technique. Can you achieve your treatment aim without positioning the arm in this way? Ultimately, causing pain increases muscle tone and is counterproductive. Some would argue that causing pain is also unethical.

Use the following tables to help you compare these techniques and help yourself to identify your preferences as you practice.

Practicing Techniques in Prone	
Technique	**My findings**
Fingers hooking 	
Fingers pushing 	
Thumbs 	

Practicing Techniques in Prone	
Technique	**My findings**
Web of hand	
Side of hand	
Forearm	

TIP: Address "tight" spots accurately. Often, the levator scapulae is very tight, inserting at the superior angle of the scapula, a point some therapists confuse with rhomboid minor. We know this is the case because when you massage such clients the tightness appears to increase as you slide your hand superiorly (i.e., as you access the levator scapulae) and because with kyphotic postures, the levator scapulae tends to contract to elevate the scapula as when maintaining a static position for prolonged periods. Be certain that when you apply pressure you are applying it to soft tissues and not to the bone itself.

TIP: Consider doing less frictioning to sore spots. The tight "knots" discovered by some therapists in the rhomboid area may be trigger spots, areas that refer pain elsewhere if "live." Holding static pressures to these areas, perhaps with a stretch (as in STR), is considered to be a good method of dealing with trigger spots rather than frictioning them. Ask yourself these questions: "When I friction the tight spots in rhomboid muscles do these spots really go away, or are they still there when the client returns for their next treatment?" "Is my frictioning being effective?"

TIP: Avoid causing discomfort. If, when massaging, you press too sharply on the medial border of the scapula, this causes discomfort and raises muscle tone. Muscles contract and as a result you assume they are tight and end up having to work harder to try and relax them. Clients with tight anterior deltoid and pectoral muscles (common in kyphotic postures) may find the half-Nelson position used in subscapular work is extremely uncomfortable, and, again, this may increase the tone of muscles, including that of the rhomboids.

Tip 17: **Treating Ribs**

If you believe that tension in the muscles of respiration of the costovertebral joints is a contributing factor to your client's symptoms, you may wish to consider the techniques described in this tip. There are many gentle, subtle ways to treat muscular tension and rib dysfunction. A selection is shown here which includes rebounding, springing, MFR to the anterior chest wall, and MFR to the diaphragm.

Seven techniques have been selected on the basis that they are varied. Hopefully you will practice with each of these and find some that suit your needs.

The seven selected techniques are as follows:
- Rebounding.
- Intercostal stroking.
- Thoracic holding.
- "Opening" one side of the rib cage.
- Springing.
- MFR to the anterior chest wall.
- MFR to the diaphragm.

Rebounding

Duncan (2012) describes how rebounding can be used when treating rib hump, breathing issues, and scoliosis. Standing to one side of your client, place one hand over the other, your palms against the client's lateral thorax and then lean into your client. Attempt to rock the body in a rhythmic motion by releasing your pressure but remaining in contact with your client. Work up and down both sides of the rib cage, on both left and right sides of the body. The pressure needs to be fairly firm, but it should still be comfortable for your client to receive. Note that rebounding is not the same as rocking (see Tip 22: Rocking (p. 281).

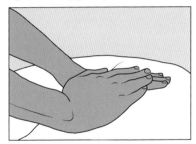

Intercostal Stroking

Where you are able to access the ribs without this being invasive, palpate gently to ascertain the intercostal spaces. Starting as medially as possible, use the pad of your thumb or a finger to gently stroke the tissues, drawing your thumb or finger laterally. This is useful when treating clients who have a tendency to sit hunched, or whose sport requires thoracic flexion—such as rowers or people using racing bikes. It is also useful when treating clients prone to spasms in this region.

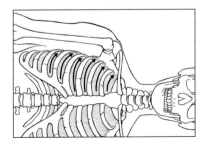

Thoracic Holding

By contrast, simply holding the thorax as shown in the illustration below is particularly relaxing and requires no movement on your part at all. Slide one hand beneath the ribs on the side of the body closest to you, place your other hand above it, and rest in this position for several minutes.

The technique can be modified to encourage deeper breathing. To do this, gently compress the ribs as your client breathes normally. Encourage your client to focus on your palm pressure and to breathe "into" your hands. As you gently reduce your pressure, the client will be encouraged to inhale more deeply in order to expand their rib cage to meet your palms.

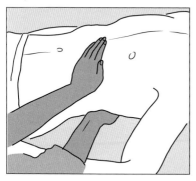

"Opening" One Side of the Rib Cage

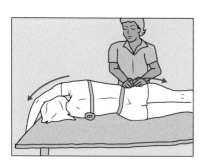

For this technique, you need to help make your client comfortable in the side-lying position, preferably with a small towel, several sponges, or a foam block beneath their thorax. Apply gentle pressure to their ilium as they take their arm over their head. If you apply gentle pressure caudally, the client will experience this mild stretch in the side of their thorax and up into their armpit. Note that this is not quite the same as a stretch for quadratus lumborum because the towel or sponge is positioned beneath the thorax not at the waist.

This technique is useful when treating clients who have been using their adductor muscles more than usual, perhaps with increased respiratory effort. An example of when this might occur is when a client has been using crutches or training hard in swimming.

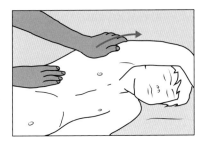

To further "open" and stretch one side of the thorax, gentle pressure can be applied in order to traction the tissues, providing this is comfortable.

Notice that the direction in which you press changes the location on the thorax where the client feels the stretch.

Springing

In Chapter 4, Tip 22: Assessing Ribs (pp. 209–210), you learned about rib springing. The technique of rib springing can be used both as an assessment and as a treatment.

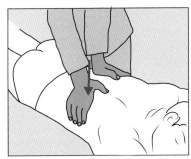

With your subject in the prone position, apply gentle pressure to the ribs one at a time to assess their "spring." Lean onto the

rib angle and then suddenly release your pressure. A tip is to assess a rib on the left and then a corresponding rib on the right, and to work your way down the body in this manner in a kind of zigzag pattern. You only need to spring each rib once or twice.

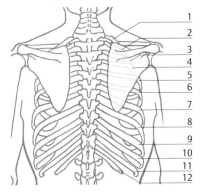

1
2
3
4
5
6
7
8
9
10
11
12

Question: Are there any contraindications to this technique?

Yes, it is contraindicated in acute conditions or in subjects suffering rheumatoid conditions or osteoporosis. Where a client has a known joint fusion such as in ankylosing spondylitis, the technique is unhelpful because the joint is fused and therefore cannot be moved.

Myofascial Release to the Anterior Chest Wall

STEP 1 Sitting to one side of the head of your treatment couch, with your client supine, place one hand so that your palm rests on the junc-tion between their neck and thorax. Place your other hand just below the sternal notch, in the midline of the body.

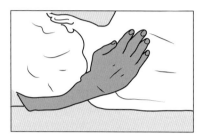

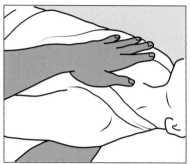

STEP 2 Using the hand that is resting on the anterior chest, apply very gentle pressure, com-pressing the chest between your hands. Be cer-tain to keep your pressure light.

As the tissues relax, you will feel your up-permost hand start to move. Follow it while maintaining contact with the skin. Where movement stops, this indicates restriction. Wait, then again follow any subsequent movement with your hand.

Note that the changes that take place during this release are subtle and require practice.

Myofascial Release to the Diaphragm

STEP 1 With your client supine, position your-self at the side of the treatment couch and place one hand over the diaphragm anteriorly and one over the diaphragm posteriorly.

STEP 2 As for MFR to the anterior chest wall, ap-ply gentle pressure with your uppermost hand, compressing your client. Notice any changes you can feel in your hands and follow in the di-rection that the tissues "pull" you, maintaining contact with the skin.

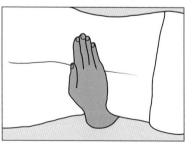

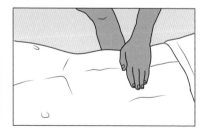

Tip 18: **Stretching the Latissimus Dorsi**

The section on "opening" the rib cage in Tip 17 (pp. 269–272) describes techniques that help stretch intercostals. The side-lying positions used for stretching the intercostals, illustrated here, also stretch the latissimus dorsi, which is a powerful arm adductor.

The latissimus dorsi can also be stretched bilaterally by elevating your client's arms above their head and applying gentle traction. Many clients feel this stretch all the way down their spine, into their sacrum. Even though this technique is shown (on the following page) being performed bilaterally, you could apply the stretch to one arm at a time.

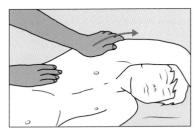

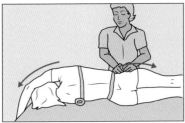

STEP 1 With your client supine, elevate their arms and hold these inferior to the elbow. Depending on the height of your couch, the client could hold your legs or waist, but some therapists may feel that this is too intimate a treatment position and therefore not appropriate for all clients.

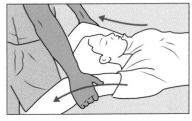

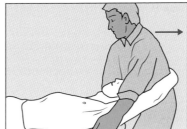

STEP 2 Gently traction the client's arms, stretching through the latissimus dorsi and the shoulder adductor muscles. If the client is holding you, the stretch is easier to apply because you simply lean back slightly. You need to practice with varying the height of your treatment table in order to find a comfortable position to traction. Hold the stretch position for around 15 seconds and release.

Question: Are there any contraindications to this stretch?

This is contraindicated for clients with shoulder subluxation or dislocation. It needs to be used with caution when treating clients with known shoulder impingement syndromes as the position of elevation could aggravate their condition. It can also be uncomfortable for clients with acromioclavicular joint problems.

Tip 19: Massage with Client on a Bolster

This simple repositioning of your client helps when treating clients who are kyphotic or with tight pectorals. In supine, ensure that their head is also supported as you place a bolster or rolled-up towel along the length of the thorax.

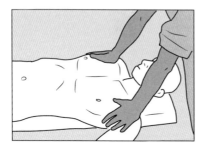

Notice when you practice this with a colleague and are receiving treatment that not only do you experience a stretch in your pectoral muscles, but also that the stretch of the pectorals feels more intense in this position.

As a therapist, you can apply various techniques including the following:

- Simple pectoral stretch, by resting on the anterior shoulder.
- Gently pressing or massaging the pectorals.
- Treating trigger spots.

When addressing trigger points in the pectorals with your client in this position, note that localized pressure, always more sensitive to receive than pressure spread over a wider area with a palm or forearm, will feel even more intense—so be cautious.

One of the disadvantages of using this position is that there is a tendency for your client to roll to one side, off the bolster, if you press down on one side only. This is usually overcome by the fact that much less pressure is required due to the heightened sensitivity of the tissues which are tractioned at the shoulder in this position.

Tip 20: **Addressing Trigger Points in the Thorax**

Trigger points can be found throughout the thorax, anteriorly in the pectoralis major and the pectoralis minor, and the abdominals, laterally in the serratus anterior, and posteriorly in the trapezius, the latissimus dorsi, and the extensor muscles. Getting your client to lie on a bolster, as described in Tip 19 (p. 274), produces an excellent position in which to palpate for trigger points in pectoral muscles because in this position the muscles are lengthened and under slight tension and only the lightest of fingertip touch is ever needed to discover a trigger point in these muscles.

One *tip* if you are new to finding trigger points is to start from a known bony landmark and to work in relation to this. For example, practice finding trigger points in your own pectorals by locating one of your clavicles. Gently run your fingertip from the lateral end of the clavicle at the shoulder (a) to the medial end, at the sternoclavicular joint (b). Try to run your fingertip inferior to the clavicle but so that you are still touching it. Notice how the gully in which you are running your fingertip becomes shallower as you near your sternum, due to the outward curve of the ribs. Do the same on your other side. Is there any difference? Did you notice any tender spots as your drew your fingertips across your chest? Next, repeat the process, but this time come a little more distal, maybe a fingertip's width lower down. Draw your fingertip lateral to medial, palpating for tender spots. Once you feel confident palpating for triggers in this manner, practice on a colleague or client either in the supine position or with them resting on a bolster as in Tip 19.

An alternative position in which to treat a client with trigger points in their pectorals is with the client sitting or reclining. Stand behind them and draw your fingertips across the muscles as if the client were supine.

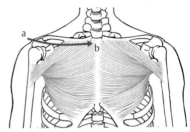

With gentle pressure on the spot, you can rest here until any discomfort dissipates or you can passively abduct your client's arm so as to slightly stretch the pectoral muscle. Some therapists ask the client to move their own arm, but this engages the pectoral muscle and you may not wish to do this.

Another area where you could practice with trigger spots is in the latissimus dorsi. With your client prone, gently palpate the muscle and when you locate a tender spot, simply grip the muscle between your fingers. Maintain your pressure until the discomfort dissipates. Alternatively, grip or compress the tender spot and ask your client to abduct their arm, thus stretching the muscle.

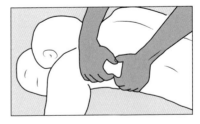

Tip 21: **Taping the Thorax**

Taping is becoming increasingly popular with the development of different types of tape. Many claims are now being made with regard to the function and effectiveness of taping. Some types of taping are designed to prevent movement of tissues (or joints), whereas others are applied with the intention of allowing—or even sometimes facilitating—movement.

One example of when a tape might be applied to the thorax to prevent movement is where a client has a single painful segment of the spine due to muscle spasming. Taping can help "offload" this region, and the principle is simply to bring the tissues together so that they are not tensioned in any way.

Another example of when you might wish to apply restrictive tape is when someone has a painful intercostal, perhaps following a tear. As with the spine, your purpose would be to limit movement in some of the soft tissues. Tape is best applied with the arm adducted—to prevent tensioning the intercostal muscles—but in practice this is difficult because in order to access the region your client needs to abduct their arm. Extending the arm as shown can facilitate access to this region.

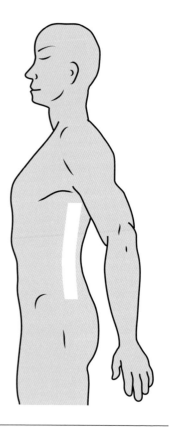

TRICK: A trick here is to have your client lying on their nonpainful side when you apply the tape.

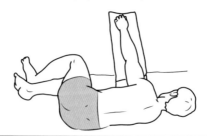

You might also wish to use a less restrictive method of taping to help improve posture. With your client in a relaxed but "good" upright posture, there are many ways to apply tape. A common and easy method is simply to create a large cross shape on the thorax, beginning at the acromion and drawing your tape posteriorly to attach to the lower ribs on the opposite side of the body.

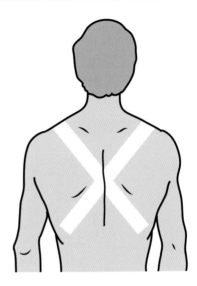

Flexible tape may be applied in a myriad of ways but should always be applied not in the neutral position but with the spine flexed and shoulders protracted. With flexible tape the "wrinkles" that appear when a client stands upright are a desired effect, and manufacturers claim this is conducive to the therapeutic process.

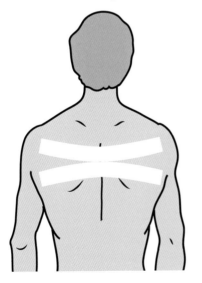

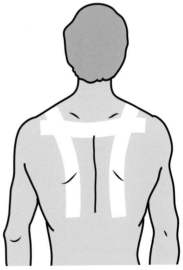

Experimenting with the Effects of Tape on the Thorax

A fun experiment you can try is to work with a colleague and practice how it feels to "wear" tapes of different patterns. A very simple exercise is to have tape applied directly over your spine while you are standing in a neutral position and to maintain this position for an hour to see how this feels. On another day, see how it feels to wear tape in the same location, but of shorter length.

Tape shape	Comments
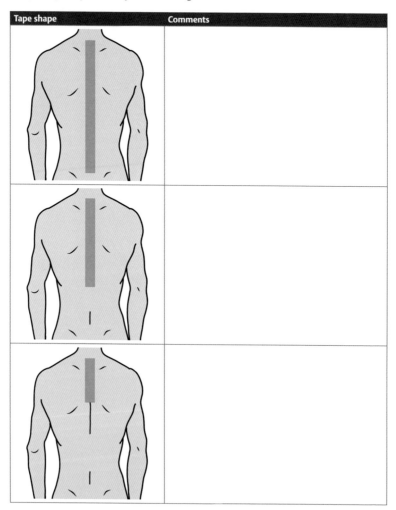	

You can experiment in this manner with all tape shapes. If you are experimenting with the simple cross shape, what effect does it have positioning the center of your cross over a different thoracic vertebra?

Tape shape	Comments

If you are using a **V** shape, have the pinnacle of the **V** end over a different vertebra. What effect does that have?

Tape shape	Comments

Tip 22: **Rocking**

In Tip 18 you learned about rebounding as a possible treatment for rib dysfunction. Rocking is similar to, but not the same as, rebounding. Rocking is a general technique which you may already have learned if you are trained as a massage therapist. Some therapists incorporate it at the start of their treatment session to relax muscles; others decide to leave it out as they vary their routines and add other skills.

To rock your client, stand to one side of your treatment couch and place one hand on your client's scapula and another on their lower ribs. Using your palms, gently push your client away from you and then roll them toward you. Like rebounding, this is a rhythmic motion, but unlike rebounding, which can be vigorous, rocking is gentle. Notice how, if you place your hands as described, your client is rocked away from you and back again rather like the trunk of a tree, whereas if you place your hand only on the client's scapula when you rock, only the top part of the thorax is moved and the pelvis remains relatively still. The effect of this is to bring about a gentle torsion in the spine, which could help with relaxing and "releasing" paraspinal muscles. Sometimes it is these very subtle techniques that prove to be effective over and above other more vigorous, forceful techniques.

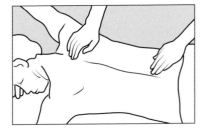

Question: How fast should I rock my client?

Fritz (2005) suggests that you attune your rocking to your client's own body rhythms and to do this you could take your client's pulse and provide rocking to match it.

Tip 23: **Varying Your Techniques**

It is easy to get stuck in a rut with your treatments, especially if you are very busy or if you lack the confidence to try new ways of working. This chapter has provided you with a variety of techniques, some of which may already be familiar to you, while others may be new, which are listed below.

- Techniques to encourage movement:
  - Thoracic expansion – Tip 2 (pp. 221–222).
  - Rocking spinous processes – Tip 3 (pp. 223–225).
  - Rib springing – Tip 17 (p. 275).
  - Rocking – Tip 22 (p. 281).
- Localized stretches and releases:
  - Longitudinal stretches, for midline spinal tissues – Tip 8 (pp. 232–233).
  - **S** strokes, for midline tissues – Tip 9 (pp. 234–235).
  - Transverse stretching – Tip 10 (p. 238).
  - Myofascial **J** strokes – Tip 12 (p. 245).
  - MFR for lateral spinal bends – Tip 12 (p. 247).
- Stillness and holding:
  - Stillness – Tip 10 (p. 237).
  - Holding – Tip 17 (p. 270).
- Compressive techniques:
  - Compression – Tip 10 (p. 237).
  - Static pressure – Tip 11 (p. 243).
  - MFR compressive technique – Tip 12 (p. 246).
  - Trigger points – Tip 20 (p. 275).
- Pressure and stretch techniques:
  - Pressure and stretch – Tip 10 (p. 238).
  - STR – Tip 13 (pp. 250–254).
- Gross MFR release:
  - Cross hand – Tip 12 (pp. 245–246).
- Stripping:
  - Stripping – Tip 10 (p. 239).
- Rolling and rocking techniques:
  - MFR thorax – Tip 12 (pp. 247–249).
  - Rebounding – Tip 17 (p. 269).

- Gross passive stretches:
  - Passive stretches – Tip 14 (pp. 255–258).
  - MET – Tip 15 (pp. 259–261).
  - Rib opening – Tip 17 (pp. 269–271); Tip 18 (p. 273).
  - Taping – Tip 21 (pp. 276–280).

For further variety, you might also like to try the following additional techniques. Again, some of them may be new to you or they may serve as reminders of earlier training you may have done.

Skin pulling: This is used to stretch soft tissues locally, helping to prevent adhesions. Without oil or wax, gently grip the skin and draw it toward you. Try to avoid pinching. Note areas that differ in skin pliability, comparing left and right side of the thorax. You may find that it is easier to pick up skin on some clients than on others, and on some clients, it cannot be pinched at all.

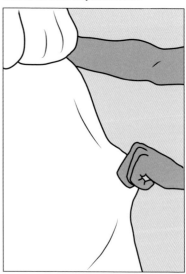

Pawing: This technique, used to relax a client and loosen soft tissues locally, can also be effective for relating one part of the body to another. Using gentle, gripping-like motions in a rhythmic manner, "paw" your way up and down your client's back either directly over the skin, without using any oil or wax, or through clothing or a towel. Keep your movements slow, controlled, and rhythmic, working at a pace that feels comfortable for you, one hand at a time, in exactly the same manner as a cat paws a cushion when it is happy.

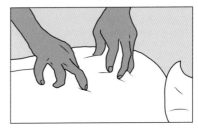

Question: Does it matter how much skin I "paw" or where I start?

How much skin you are able to draw up with your fingertips will vary between clients. It does not matter where you start. You could start at the lumbar spine on one side of the spine and paw your way to the neck, then at the neck change sides and paw your way down the other side of the body to the lumbar spine. Once there, retrace your steps back to your start position.

Skin compression: This is useful to decrease tone locally and to facilitate circulation through gentle compression and relaxation of the skin and underlying tissues. Check pliability both before and after employing this technique, using the techniques described in Chapter 4. Starting anywhere that feels appropriate, gently draw the skin together for a second or two and release. You can repeat, or move to a new spot about a thumb's width away, covering a small area. Notice how the area quickly reddens as blood flow is stimulated and how the pliability of tissues improves. You can use oil or a massage medium, but greater traction on tissues is achieved without it.

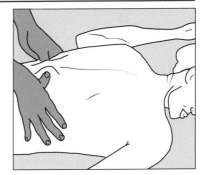

Digital pressure: This technique is useful to deactivate trigger spots or to address an increase in tone locally. It can also be used on areas that are cramping. Most therapists learn to use fingers in their training but sometimes fall back on using their thumbs. Reinforcing your fingers as shown in the illustration below allows you to save your thumb joints and does not require a lot of pressure to bring about a change in soft tissues. You can use your fingers to maintain pressure on a spot, or to apply gentle transverse stretches of the skin, pushing it away from you. Notice that if you rub your fingertips back and forth across a muscle as is sometimes advocated, this can be irritating for the long extensor muscles of the thorax, which sometimes react with an increase, rather than a decrease, in tone.

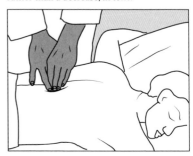

Tapotement: This is a useful technique for when you wish to increase tone in a muscle and stimulate blood flow. It can be useful at the end of a session to help "wake up" a client, provided it is done subtly so as not to "jolt" them awake. Hacking, using ulnar border/little finger (a), cupping, with cupped palms (b), and pummeling, with loose fists (c) are all excellent variations on a theme.

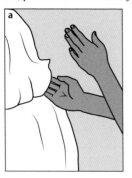
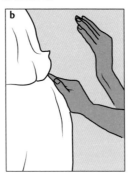
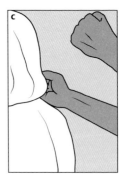

Forearms for compression, gliding, brushing, stretching: Many therapists develop problems with their wrists, fingers, and thumbs due to overuse, so it is good to get into the habit of limiting use of your hands where possible. Consider using your forearms for some techniques. You can use your forearm on dry skin to stimulate blood flow and create warmth by rubbing one or both arms over the back of your subject; you can lean through one or both forearms to apply gentle compression of tissues (remember to avoid pressure to vertebrae themselves or to the scapulae); with oil, you can use your forearms to help glide across the back of the body or to pin and stretch tissues.

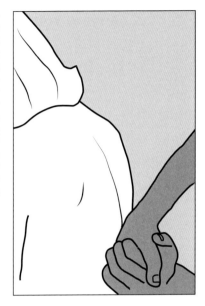

Tip 24: **Changing Your Treatment Position**

This final treatment tip is a reminder that you can alter your treatment position. If you are an experienced therapist, changing position may be second nature to you. However, newly qualified or student therapists tend to consider this less often, which is understandable: once you have a client in a comfortable position, it seems unproductive to move them. Even therapists who have been practicing for quite a while sometimes get into a rut and in some instances where you have been slow to progress a treatment and resolve a client's problem, it is worth discussing different treatment positions with them. Practicing with a colleague will help you to become adept at moving clients with the least amount of fuss, maintaining correct towel draping, and reestablishing a sequence. Where a client comes to you with a very specific problem, it is often useful to try different approaches on different visits. Sometimes a technique that does not work particularly well in one position works excellently in another. Throughout this chapter, different treatment positions have been illustrated. Over the next few pages, some of these illustrations are presented again, grouped by position, with reminders as to their uses.

Prone: This is one of the most common treatment positions when treating clients with thoracic problems. Remember that you can passively retract the scapula by placing something beneath the shoulder.

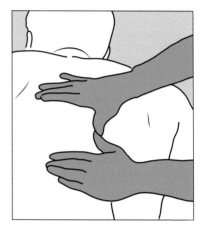

Remember also that you can work from the side of the couch to rock the client's body or to rock individual spinous processes and to work transversely across tissues.

Supine: This is another common treatment position and is useful for addressing issues in the clavicle and pectoral muscle. Remember that you can modify the position by placing a bolster or towel longitudinally beneath your client, remembering to support their head.

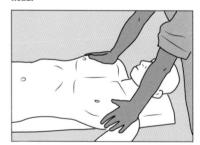

Remember, too, that you can also use this position when treating lower ribs and the diaphragm, and you can modify the position so that your client is semi-recumbent.

Seated: This position is useful when encouraging thoracic expansion, when treating the upper pectorals, or when applying techniques to the erector spinae muscles.

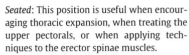

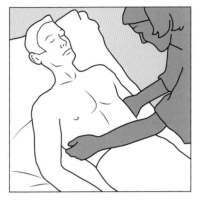

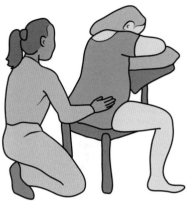

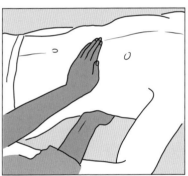

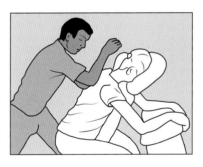

Side lying: This position is useful for "opening" the uppermost side of the rib cage and for permitting techniques to the intercostals on that side of the latissimus dorsi, and rhomboids (through scapular stretching).

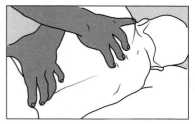

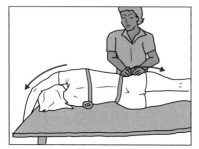

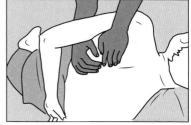

Chapter VI

Thoracic Aftercare

Chapter 6 **Thoracic Aftercare**

The aftercare tips in this chapter include chest stretches and breathing exercises, the self-treatment of trigger points, postural correction, and techniques to overcome spasm in the muscle of the thorax. There are of course some important stretches for the upper back too, with guidelines for how these should be carried out. As with the aftercare advice in other chapters, you could use this information to either create a generic handout for your clients or tailor it to their specific needs. Get feedback from them on which aspects of aftercare are useful.

Not everything will work for all clients. In this manner, you can start to build up your own unique database of tips and tricks for the thoracic region and may even start to come up with your own ideas. Many of the tips included in this book were gleaned from years of working with clients during which I kept notes about what they said they did to treat their own back problems. At that time, some of these were not well known, yet have since become popularized, for example, the self-management of trigger points and some of the back stretches.

Tip 1: Ten Chest Stretches

When providing aftercare for clients with thoracic problems, chest stretches are valuable for four reasons:

- First, one of the problems commonly encountered in clients with thoracic pain is "poor" posture. This usually describes the kind of posture where a person has "rounded" shoulders, their head craned too far forward, not balanced over their thorax. Clients with such postures have lengthened rhomboid muscles due to protraction of the scapulae, and shortened pectorals. Holding a chest stretched for around 30 seconds daily is likely to result in improved posture.
- Second, stretches such as those described here can help some clients with breathing problems by "opening" the chest region, increasing thoracic expansion.
- Third, they can help reduce pain in both chest and upper back muscles.
- Finally, changing the shape of the thorax helps clients to reposition their head and this often reduces neck pain. In some cases, it reduces pain in the lower back too.

Ten stretches illustrated on the following pages range from the simple (stretches 1, 2, 3, and 4) to the more advanced (5, 6, 7, and 8) and specific (9 and 10) stretches. Experiment with these examples, selecting those you think are appropriate for your clients.

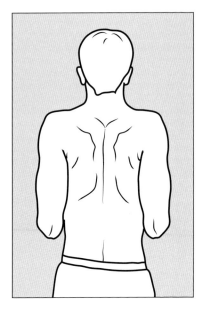

Stretch 1 As rhomboid muscles are the antagonists to the pectorals, simply contracting rhomboids helps reduce tone in pectorals.

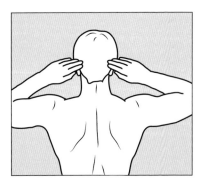

Stretch 2 A *trick* is to ask a client simply to touch the back of their head as shown alongside. In performing this action, they contract rhomboids. The pectorals are stretched if, once in this position, your subject takes their elbows backward.

Stretch 3 This stretch can be modified by holding the hands behind the back. Not everyone can do this, however.

Stretch 4 A towel could be used. Notice how varying the position of the towel varies the location in the chest muscle where the stretch is experienced.

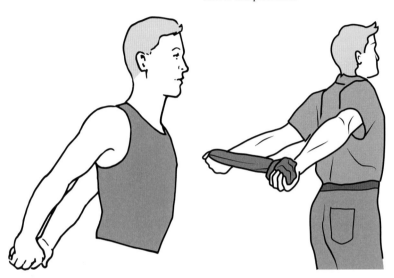

Question: Are there any contraindications to these stretches?

Extending the arms in this way with a towel is contraindicated for clients with a history of shoulder subluxations or dislocations.

When a client has space and time available, the following two chest stretches could be used.

Stretch 5 The client rests in the supine position with a towel rolled up and placed lengthwise down the thorax. The head also needs support, either with this towel or with a pillow; otherwise, it falls back, extending the neck and this can be uncomfortable. The advantage of using a towel is that it can be folded or rolled to suit the size of the client. The disadvantage is that heavier clients may need something stronger against which to rest.

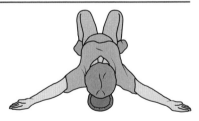

A bolster or foam roller can be used instead of a towel, but some clients find it difficult to position themself on the roller and, of course, the length of the roller cannot be adjusted.

Stretch 6 Standing with their back to a wall, a client could try to press the back of their arms into the wall, using different arm positions, from horizontal to elevated. Alternatively, they could squat, thus changing the position of their arms in that way.

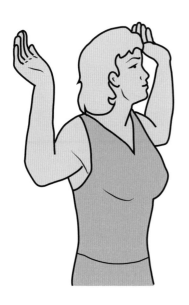

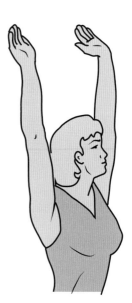

Stretch 7 Where a client has the edge of a wall available, they could stand close to the wall and experiment with stretching different fibers of their pectoralis major muscles by altering the position of their arms.

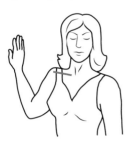

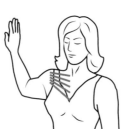

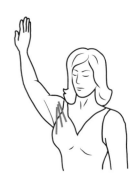

Stretch 8 Where a doorway is available, the same stretch can be performed as the client steps "into" the doorway, varying the arm position as illustrated under stretch 7.

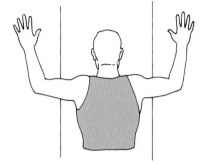

Stretches 9 and 10 There are various ways of stretching the pectoral muscles, and it can be fun to give a client the challenge of experimenting and discovering for themselves the positions they find most effective. They could utilize something they have close to hand such as a chair (stretch 9), wall, or a park bench, or they could simply alter their position. A client who is bedbound could stretch simply by pushing themselves upward (stretch 10).

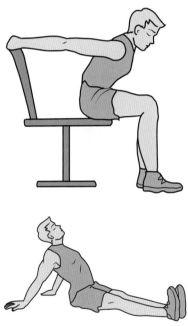

Tip 2: **Eight Upper Back Stretches**

Stretches to the upper part of the back are particularly useful for helping to decrease pain resulting from muscle tension in this region of the spine. They are particularly useful for clients who maintain static postures for long periods of time as part of their work or hobbies and can be used both to relieve the pain of muscle tension once it occurs and, prophylactically, on a regular basis throughout the day for 30 seconds in order to decrease the likelihood of tension developing.

A selection of upper back stretches has been provided here and, as for chest stretches, these range from the simple (stretches 1, 2, 3, and 4) to the more advanced (5, 6, 7, and 8) stretches.

Stretch 1 In the hug position, the scapulae protract and the rhomboids are lengthened. To enhance the stretch, instruct your client to adopt this position and then to take their chin to their chest.

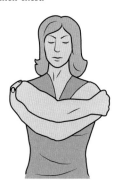

Stretch 2 Rounding the back while standing or sitting, pushing the back upward, also stretches the rhomboid muscles.

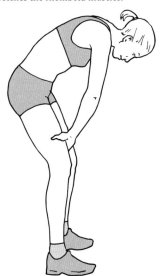

Stretch 3 An alternative, which also stretches the thoracic erector spinae, is to round the back with head and neck flexion. Be careful not to place too much force on the head and neck in this position.

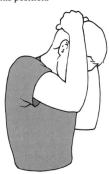

A disadvantage of these positions is possible cramp in the abdominals, which are shortened and, especially in stretch 2, actively engaged.

Stretch 4 This is similar to stretch 2 but is performed in the kneeling position. As with stretch 2, the client needs to focus on contracting their abdominals in order to arch their back. It is sometimes referred to as a "cat stretch."

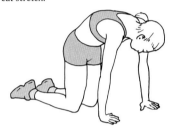

Stretch 5 Stretch 1 could be enhanced by grasping the sides of a chair and then leaning gently backward. Caution is needed for clients with a history of shoulder subluxation or dislocation.

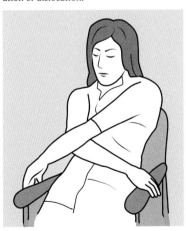

Stretch 6 Simply hanging from a rope with one or both arms in front of the body stretches the rhomboids. Again, caution is needed when used for clients with a history of shoulder subluxation or dislocation.

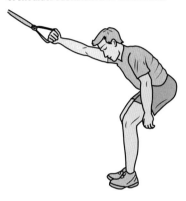

Stretch 7 Leaning forward in a chair and hooking the hand beneath a foot provides a good anchor to stretch one set of rhomboids at a time. It does, however, require the flexibility for rotation, which not all clients possess.

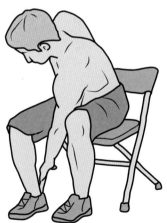

Stretch 8 Alternatives are simply to lean forward and reach beneath the chair or hook the hands around or beneath the feet.

Caution: Stretches 7 and 8 are contraindicated in clients with a previous history of disk herniations. Overweight clients may find it uncomfortable to squash their chest and abdomen in this way.

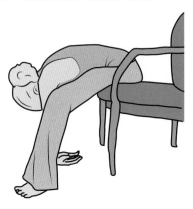

Tip 3: Self-treatment of Trigger Points in the Thorax

Trigger points, localized points of palpable tenderness, are found throughout the thorax, including around the medial border of the scapulae between approximately T4 and T6 (a), close to the spine itself in deep rotatores (b), within the longitudinal extensor muscles (c), and in the pectoralis minor (d) and the pectoralis major (e) muscles.

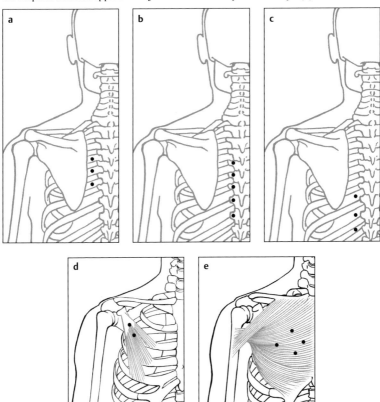

You can help your client to treat these sore spots in their muscles by teaching them how to use a ball safely to apply gentle pressure to the point for a minute or two daily.

Question: Are there any contraindications to self-treating triggers in this way?

Yes, clients who bruise easily or with fragile skin or osteoporosis should avoid self-triggering as they risk harm to their bones and soft tissues due to the very localized point of pressure these techniques employ.

Simple ways to self-trigger posterior points are to place a tennis ball or a firm therapy ball between the back and a wall (a). Crossing the arms (b) protracts the scapulae, enabling your client to access their rhomboids with the muscles in a lengthened position.

TIP: Placing the ball inside a long sock and holding it over one shoulder means that the client will not have to keep bending down to pick up the ball each time it falls when they attempt to alter their standing position.

An alternative is for the client to lie on a ball (c).

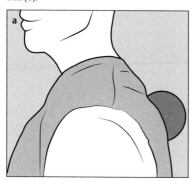

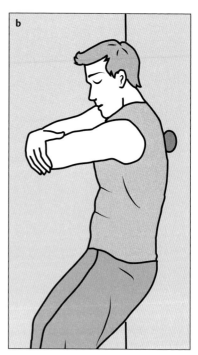

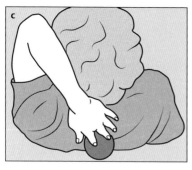

Trigger points in chest muscles can be treated similarly. The gentlest approach is to hold a ball to the trigger point (a). For deeper pressure, the client can gently press their chest to a ball positioned against a wall (b).

Taking an arm into extension (c) provides a form of active soft tissue release, stretching the tissues in which the trigger point is housed.

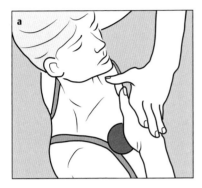

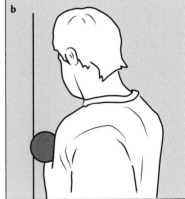

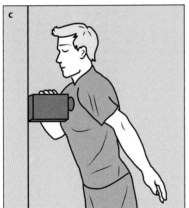

Tip 4: Thoracic Expansion Exercises

Different exercises are likely to produce expansion in different parts of the thorax. In the study by Paulin et al (2003), the subjects all had COPD (chronic obstructive pulmonary disease) and after performing the exercises like those shown on the following pages demonstrated an expansion of the inferior region of the thorax. As a variety of exercises was used, it is not clear whether there was one specific exercise responsible for improving the thoracic expansion or whether they were all equally effective. Other studies have shown that exercise can increase the apical portion of the thorax. What is interesting is that the exercises listed by Paulin et al involve improving thoracic mobility through flexion, extension, and rotation exercises, all of them movements that are easy for a client to perform at home and

therefore could be a useful addition to your intervention as a therapist.

Extension of the thorax is encouraged by leaning backward while standing (a) or sitting (b), and can be enhanced by placing a small pillow or rolled-up towel between the thoracic region and a chair. Resting in the sphinx position (c) or extending the elbows (d), as shown, is also useful. Resting on the knees with arms elevated (e) stretches the chest and helps improve extension. Use of a foam roller (f) has also been advocated, but note that this requires the weight of a client's own body to roll up and down on the roller and it is quite a severe exercise, contraindicated for clients with low bone density or arthritic conditions. It is also inappropriate for clients with scoliosis and may be difficult or even painful for clients with kyphosis.

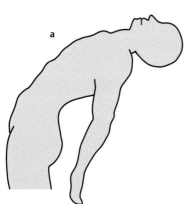

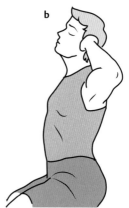

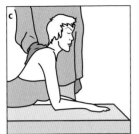

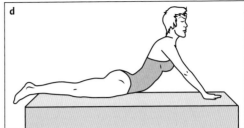

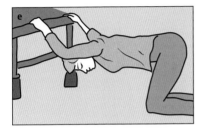

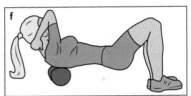

Rotation of the thorax is encouraged by sitting in a chair and rotating with the arms crossed (a), holding the seat of a chair to facilitate this movement (b), and side bends to encourage lateral flexion (c).

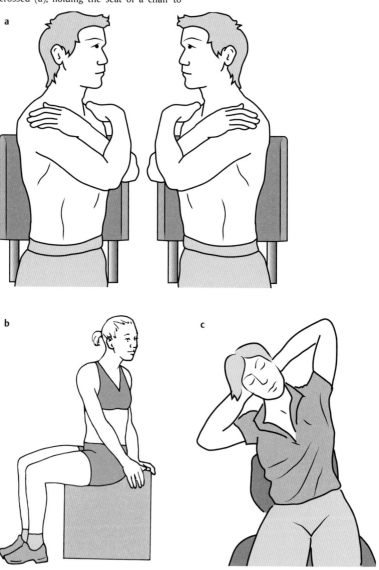

Flexion of the thorax is encouraged by movements that round the upper back. Most clients do not need to encourage thoracic flexion because many have kyphotic type postures. However, clients with thoracic "flat back" benefit from improving flexion in this region of their spine as part of a thoracic expansion program.

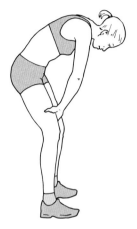

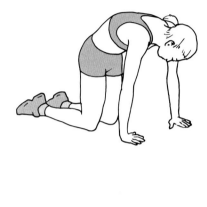

Does It Work?

If you are curious to know whether these exercises help in increasing thoracic expansion, you could try an experiment for yourself. You could begin by measuring a subject's thoracic excursion, using the information in Chapter 4, Tip 15 (pp. 00–00). Then identify whether you think your subject has a reduced range of movement into flexion, extension, or rotation. Select one or more of the exercises shown here to be performed regularly. Document the date and your initial excursion measurement, and which range of movement is restricted, which exercises you have given your client, how often you have asked them to perform the exercise (twice daily, for example). After 7 days, measure excursion again. Did your selected protocol help your client to improve their thoracic expansion? Which factors do you think contributed to the success (or failure) of your experiment?

Subject name: _____

	Date	Date
Thoracic excursion measurement		
Most reduced range of movement (flexion, extension, or rotation)		

Exercises selected: _____
Number of times these were performed daily: _____

Tip 5: Breathing Exercises

There are many different exercises that may be used to improve breathing. Section 2 of the book is aimed at massage therapists and general body workers, so the exercises that have been selected are simple and useful in helping to stretch soft tissues and muscles, including the intercostals, perhaps following a muscle tear, or for rib fracture in the post-acute stages. On the next few pages, you will find four simple exercises:

• Exercise A: Simple rib expansion.
• Exercise B: Upper or lower rib expansion.
• Exercise C: Unilateral rib stretch.
• Exercise D: Rib and intercostal mobilizer.

These have been adapted from the exercises described by Berry (1963) for the rehabilitation of soldiers with chest injuries. They are not intended to be performed in any particular order, but are provided as good examples of simple, useful exercises.

Exercise A: Simple Rib Expansion

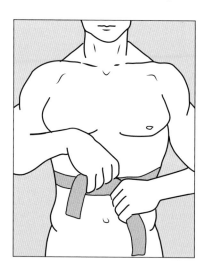

To encourage overall rib expansion, your client places a piece of tape or a tape measure around their chest and practices inhaling two or three times, pushing their chest against the tape. If they use an actual tape measure, they can observe and even record the measurements. Some clients find this motivating. Note that your client may practice this twice a day, but it is important that they only inhale two or three times on each session to prevent fatigue and also to prevent becoming lightheaded. Compare this to Chapter 5, Tip 2: Encouraging Thoracic Expansion (pp. 221–222).

Exercise B: Upper or Lower Rib Expansion

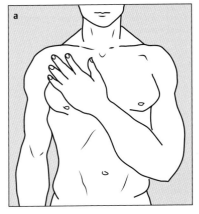

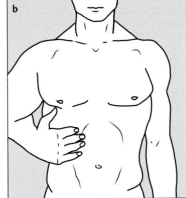

In this exercise, your client places their hand on the upper or lower ribs in order to encourage rib expansion on a particular side and of a particular part of their chest. Where they place their hand is where they are going to focus their attention on. They breathe in as much air as possible and then use their hand to help push air out as they exhale. Repeat just two or three times.

TIP: Observing the movement of the hand by looking at it directly or in a mirror helps to reinforce movement of the rib cage in that region.

Exercise C: Unilateral Rib Stretch

To stretch a previously injured side, instruct your client to inhale as they gently raise their arm into abduction and up into elevation. At the maximum point of elevation, your client holds this position for a few seconds before lowering their arm and repeating once or twice more.

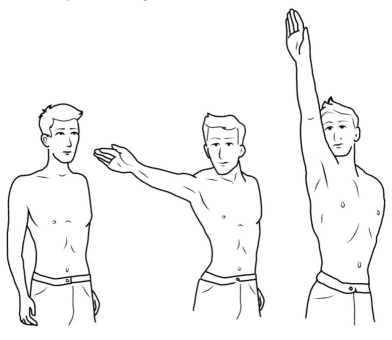

TIP: If your client finds it difficult to inhale deeply as they perform this movement, suggest that they perform it while breathing normally. This in itself stretches the soft tissues on the injured side.

Exercise D: Rib and Intercostal Mobilizer

In this slightly more difficult exercise, your client presses their hand against the side that is *uninjured* and reinforces this with their other hand. The elbow on the affected side is held slightly away from the body.

They inhale and then rotate toward the uninjured side, leading with their shoulder. Once they have rotated, they exhale strongly and return to the start position.

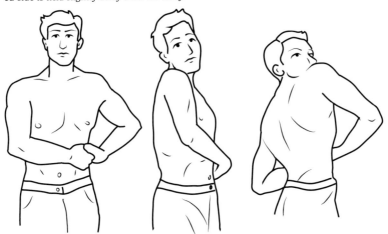

For example, if dysfunction in the thorax is on the right, the subject places both hands on their ribs on the left. They hold their right elbow away from their body while maintaining contact with their right hand against the left side of the thorax. They inhale, and rotate to the left. Once rotated to the left, they exhale strongly and then return to the start position.

Tip 6: Improving Daily Posture

One of reasons people experience musculoskeletal thoracic pain is due to their maintaining a static posture for prolonged periods of time. It is as fatiguing to try and maintain a forced, erect posture as it is to remain slouched. Although an upright posture held for a long period of time is preferable to a slouched posture, it can also lead to pain. Bodies like movement and one of the best ways to overcome postural strain is to change position from one posture to another. You can help your client to do this by first helping them to identify those occasions when they might be retaining a posture for a long time.

Start by asking your client to identify how long they spend in any of these postures, over a 24-hour period. "Combination" postures are those that are neither standing nor sitting. For example, a gas engineer may spend most of their day squatting on one or both legs to check gas meters; a car mechanic may spend time standing in the pit beneath a car with their head and neck in extension and their arms elevated while they repair the underside of a vehicle.

Next, look at the table on the next page and the suggestions provided for overcoming this static posture.

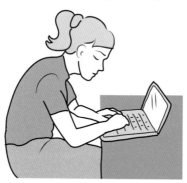

Posture	Time spent in 24 h
Standing	
Sitting	
Lying	
In combination postures related to work	
In combination postures related to a hobby	
Any other types of posture held for a long period of time	

Prolonged posture	Ways to alleviate this posture
Standing	• Sit when possible—for example, if standing is part of your job, make a point of sitting during breaks • Stretch your arms above your head • Hug one knee at a time • Perform pelvic tilts • Perform hip hitches • Deliberately protract and then retract your shoulders • Lean down to one side a little, and then to the other • Twist to one side and then to the other
Sitting	• Stand whenever possible • If you find yourself leaning forward, make an effort to lean backward • Hug one knee and then the other • Change how you sit. For example, if you are slouching for a long period, sit upright • Lift one buttock off the chair and then the other • If you sit cross-legged, sit with your legs uncrossed • Protract and then retract your shoulders
Combination postures	• Wherever possible, take a few minutes to put your body into the opposite posture to that of the prolonged posture • Alternate which side of the body you use if that is possible. If you squat on your left leg, try squatting on your right leg • Wherever possible, request a workstation assessment

How does your client feel about the suggestions made in the table above for preventing static posture? Could your client incorporate any of these into their routine? What other ways can you think of to help your client change position? Better still, what suggestions does your client have?

Sometimes, it is hard to avoid prolonged postures. For example, a person may be obliged to stand for a long time on a train in order to commute.

It may seem challenging when a client learns that they might need to change a routine that has become habitual. Identifying prolonged periods of immobility is a key starting point. By identifying these postures, your client is acknowledging that they may be contributing to thoracic pain, and once this seed is sewn in your client's mind, he or she is much more likely to find their own ways of overcoming poor posture.

Tip 7: **Overcoming Spasm**

Spasm in the thoracic region commonly occurs in the abdominals, usually when we adopt a prolonged posture of trunk flexion and/or rotation.

Ways to overcome muscle spasm include the following, as shown in the illustration below:

- Stretching the affected muscle (a) and (b).
- Static pressures to the affected muscle (c).
- Isometric contraction or concentric contraction of opposing muscle group (d).
- Static pressure *and* stretch to the affected muscle. Here the client might press into

their muscle and either lean backward or rotate to the opposite side.

- Positional release technique. Here the client finds the most comfortable resting position, often shortening the muscle. Positional release can be achieved actively but is more effective if used by a therapist.

It is worthwhile chatting to your client to see if they can identify key postures that trigger spasm so that they can avoid these where possible.

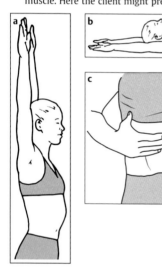
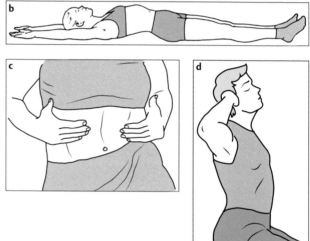

Tip 8: Help for Scoliosis

It is beyond the scope of this section to detail the treatments for scoliosis. However, corrective exercise, under supervision and with regular reassessment, can help. Very generally, a client attempts to lengthen shortened tissues by stretching these, and to shorten lengthened tissues by strengthening them. For example, they might use a block to reposition their pelvis while attempting to lean against a wall (a) or a resistance band while seated (b). It is important to remember that these movements activate many muscles, stabilizers as well as agonists, and a detailed knowledge of this kind of strengthening is needed before attempting to help clients with scoliotic postures.

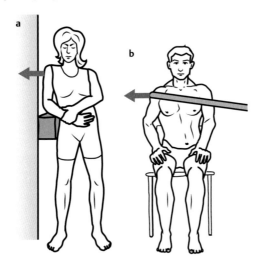

Tip 9: Muscle Strengthening Exercises

Generally, exercise is good for alleviating thoracic pain of musculoskeletal origin. Movement, of joints, ligaments, muscles, and other soft tissues, is usually beneficial unless a person has an acute injury. Simple scapular retractions as might be used to stretch the pectorals (Tip 1) help to strengthen rhomboid muscles, and activities such as rowing and rock climbing strengthen rhomboids and many others. Frequently found to be weak in subjects with poor posture are the lower fibers of the trapezius. To strengthen these, your client can perform a simple exercise sometimes referred to as the "dart" because it involves adopting a dart-shaped position.

STEP 1 Your client sits or stands and gently draws back their scapulae. This involves both rhomboid muscles and the middle fibers of the trapezius.

STEP 2 While in this position, your client then gently depresses their shoulders. One way to achieve this is to suggest to your client that they try to press their elbows to the floor (or into the arms of a chair if they are seated).

TIP: To help your clients identify the location of their lower fibers of the trapezius and to check that these are contracting, it is useful if you feel for the 12th rib and locate the 12th thoracic vertebra. If you then move your fingers slightly upward, you will be on the lowest fibers of trapezius. Gently tap this spot prior to the exercise so that your client can focus their attention on it.

This position is held for a few seconds. The aim is gradually to build up the length of time that your client can hold this low-level contraction. It is important that they do not try to maximally retract and/or depress their scapulae, as this will induce tension and fatigue and possibly soreness in the lower fibers of the trapezius.

TIP: If your client practices this exercise in the prone position, it is a little more challenging because they are retracting their scapulae against gravity in the initial part of the exercise.

Tip 10: **Other Approaches**

There are many different tools and techniques for treating clients with problems in the thoracic region. As with other parts of the spine, simple techniques include the following:

- The application of heat or cold, useful in reducing pain.
- Some clients report achieving some relief from using a transcutaneous electrical nerve stimulation (TENS) machine.
- At the more extreme end of the spectrum of tools available are inversion tables and devices designed to traction the spine, both of which require specialist knowledge for their application.

Shown on the following pages is just a small selection of devices may have come across, with a note on how each might be used:

- Balls.
- Foam rollers.
- Trigger point devices.
- Back stretchers.

Balls

Therapy balls of various sizes are used in the aftercare of clients with thoracic problems. The balls range from small balls such as tennis balls, for addressing trigger points (as you have seen on pp. 300–301), and medium-sized soft rubber balls, used to stretch the pectorals in prone position (a), to large "gym" balls frequently used to show how subjects can stretch the pectorals in the supine position (b).

a
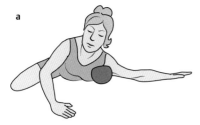

b
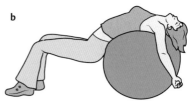

Foam Rollers

These may be used to stretch pectorals (a), or they may be used to roll up and down in order to mobilize the thoracic spine (b). Note that when using them for the purposes of mobilization, caution is needed because in the positions shown here, a lot of force is placed on the spine in a localized area, and this would be contraindicated for clients with osteoporosis or a history of disk herniation. Caution is also needed for clients with rheumatoid conditions of the spine.

a
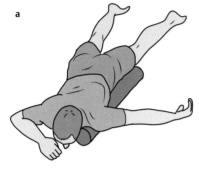

b
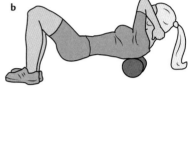

Trigger Point Devices

Trigger point devices are used to treat trigger points and include simple double-ball devices (a), plastic **S**-shaped devices (b), and all manner of curved plastic devices (c) designed to facilitate access of trigger points from any angle.

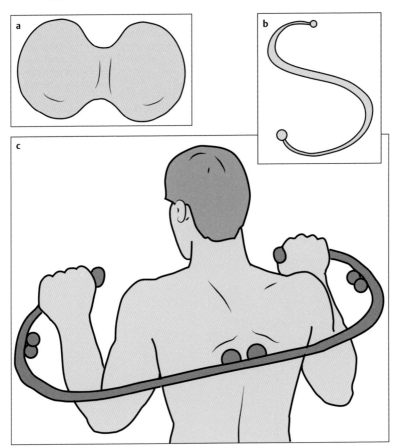

Back Stretchers

Back Stretchers are available in various lengths and designs, ranging from simple, flat, or curved products to more elaborate devices designed to fit into the erector spinae.

These are particularly useful in treating clients with kyphotic postures, but care is needed because they can result in point-specific pressure to ribs and so are contraindicated for clients with osteoporosis, and need to be used with caution in others.

There are all manner of devices, old and new, to assist in the treatment of clients with musculoskeletal problems, and it is tempting to feel the need to know how to use them all.

Experimentation is good and many devices are useful, particularly those that help a therapist safeguard their own joints.

However, it is knowledge and skills, rather than fancy devices, which are likely to be most effective for both you and your client in helping to address problems in the thoracic region. Bushcraft expert Ray Mears (1996) notes that it is knowledge of bushcraft itself, rather than a rucksack full of fancy equipment, that is important in planning expeditions because, he says, "Knowledge doesn't weigh anything." The same could be said for the world of manual therapy: even the most basic of hands-on skills and understanding can be more valuable than an expensive piece of equipment. I hope that this section of the book has given you some ideas that you can put into your therapeutic rucksack and that you will find these useful on your own ongoing journey.

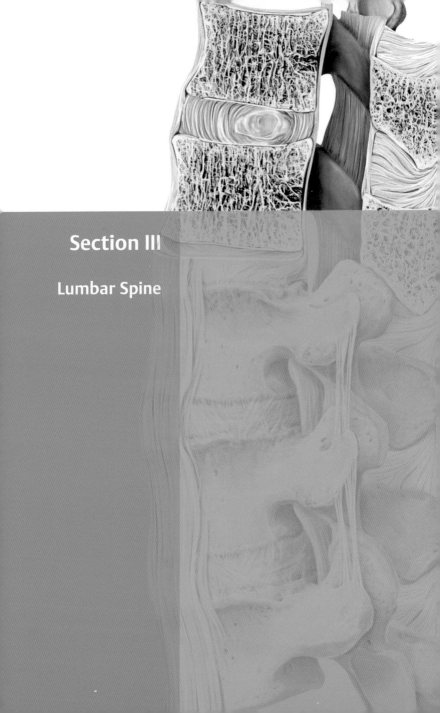

Section III

Lumbar Spine

Introduction

If you are reading this book as a therapist or as a health professional, you will no doubt be aware that for many years a huge amount of research has focused on the lumbar spine. The reason for this may be that so many people report experiencing problems in this area of their back—we all know someone who either has or has had low back pain, for example, and problems in the hip and lower limb are often attributed to dysfunction in the lumbar spine. A systematic review study by Furlan et al (2002) found that massage may be beneficial for people with chronic and nonspecific low back pain, especially when combined with exercises and education. In their evaluation of adverse effects of massage in pain-related conditions, Yin et al (2014) also carried out a systematic review and reported that massage therapies were not devoid of risks, but the incidents of such events were low. (Serious events were associated with spinal manipulation, which *The Big Back Book* does not include.) It is likely, then, that some therapists reading this book will have been using massage when treating clients and may have been getting good results.

However, we know that massage alone is not a cure for problems in the lumbar region. If it were, no one would have back pain. The material presented in this section of the book offers additional, though not necessarily alternative, treatments. Similar to the chapters on the neck and thorax, here you will find suggestions for lumbar assessment, treatment, and aftercare, which you may not yet be using. I encourage you to use these to compliment your existing practice and to share your results with colleagues and the therapeutic community as a whole.

Chapter VII

Lumbar Assessment

Chapter 7 **Lumbar Assessment**

You may have been reading this book from start to finish and if so, you will have come to realize that the assessment sections follow a similar pattern. Thirteen tips in this chapter cover the identification of bony landmarks, assessment of range of movements, and information that can be gained from palpation, but also include information on sleeping positions, the effect of daily activities on low back position, plus an example of a specialist back pain questionnaire.

When you are treating a large number of clients, it can be tempting to minimize your assessment of the lumbar region in order to get on with treatment, especially if you know your client enjoys massage or manual therapy. Yet we all know that the bodywork profession has now moved into the era of evidence-based practice and so it is important to take baseline measurements. These do not need to be extensive, nor do they need to be elaborate, but they must give you some measure of your effectiveness. The tips in this chapter offer some suggestions.

If, during the assessment, you believe that your subject may have a serious condition or a problem that is outside your scope of practice, then stop the assessment and refer them to another practitioner. Alternatively, if you have a willing colleague who is free from any low back complaints, then perhaps partner up with them to practice the assessment tips given here. You can then determine which of these tips might be most useful to you and the clients you treat.

Tip 1: Identifying Key Bony Landmarks

Let us begin this section on assessment tips for the lumbar spine by reminding ourselves about some key bony landmarks. The lumbar spine is located between the 12th thoracic vertebra (T12) and the sacrum. The five (sometimes six) vertebrae of the lumbar spine (L1–L5) have quadrate-shaped spinous processes that can be difficult to identify individually beneath the thick layer of fascia that lies over them.

Identifying the First Lumbar Vertebra

To identify the first lumbar vertebra (L1), locate the 12th thoracic vertebra and palpate inferiorly to this. The 12th thoracic vertebra is attached to the 12th rib, so it could be located by locating the 12th rib. The 11th rib, which rests almost horizontal to the 12th thoracic vertebra, is more prominent.

Identifying the Fifth Lumbar Vertebra

To identify the fifth lumbar vertebra, locate the top of the sacrum and palpate superiorly to this. It can also be difficult to differentiate between the sacrum and the spinous process of the fifth lumbar vertebra, again due to the thick layer of overlying fascia. So an alternative is to locate the fourth lumbar vertebra, which is about parallel with the iliac crest. Place your hands on the waist of your subject and press down onto their iliac crests. In this position, your thumbs will fall approximately over the fourth vertebra.

Note that there is good inter-rater reliability for palpation of the lumbar spine but poor inter-rater reliability (McKenzie and Taylor 1997), so always make your own assessment of each client you are treating rather than relying on the assessment of a colleague.

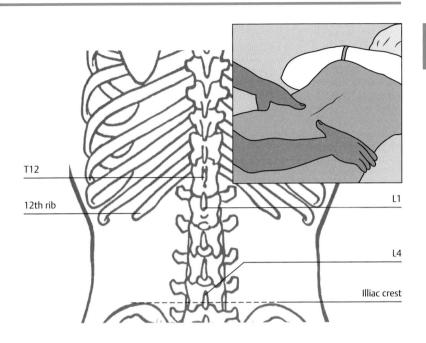

T12

12th rib

L1

L4

Illiac crest

Tip 2: Postural Assessment of the Lumbar Region

Information gained from carrying out a postural assessment of the lumbar spine can help inform your treatment. It can be easy to forget or to overlook simple things. For example, the position and depth of skin creases provide a clue to whether the pelvis is level and whether there is any lateral flexion in the spine: the deeper the crease, usually the greater the degree of flexion to that side. However, skin creases also appear when we extend. So creases can also indi-

cate increased lordosis or rotation. Test this for yourself. If you have a willing colleague with visible skin creases, stand behind them and notice that a crease will deepen when your subject extends and laterally flexes.

You will need to consider the position of the thorax also, but for now, here are some reminders to some of the things to look for when observing the lumbar spine and pelvis, and questions you may ask yourself as you carry out the assessment.

Posterior View

Does the spine appear vertical or is there any evidence of lateral curvature (a)?

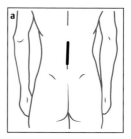

Is the lumbar musculature symmetrical or is there evidence of hypertonicity in erector spinae, for example (b)?

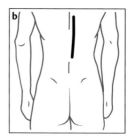

Are the iliac crests level or does one side of the pelvis seem higher than the other (c)?

Are skin creases symmetrical in height and depth?

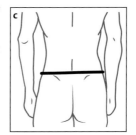

Are the posterior superior iliac spines level (d)?

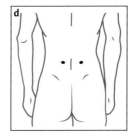

Are the ischia level? These cannot be seen, so you need to observe whether the buttock creases are level instead (e).

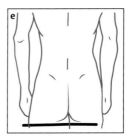

Is the pelvis in a neutral position (f) or is there evidence of clockwise (g) or anti-clockwise rotation (h)? You can assess this by asking whether one side of the pelvis appears closer to you than the other as in these pictures, which have been exaggerated for the purpose of illustration.

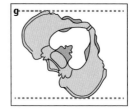

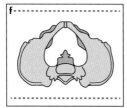

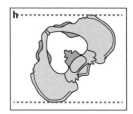

Lateral View

Does the lumbar curve appear neutral (a) or is there evidence of hyperlordosis (b) or hypolordosis (c)?

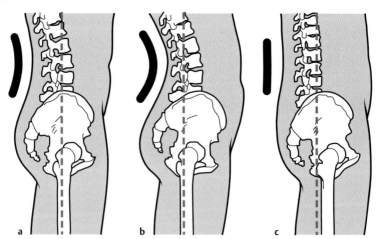

Is the abdomen flat or protruding?

Is the pelvis in a neutral position (d) or is there evidence of an anterior (e) or posterior (f) pelvic tilt?

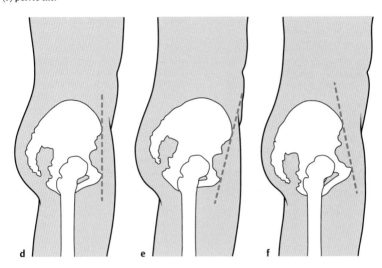

Anterior View

Is the abdomen protruding (a)?

Does the pelvis appear level (b)?

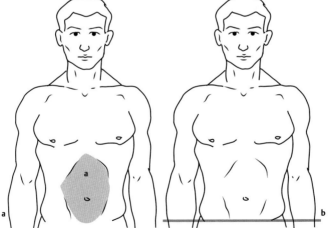

Is the pelvis in a neutral position (c) or is there any evidence of pelvic rotation clockwise (d) or anticlockwise (e)?

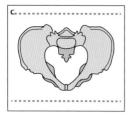

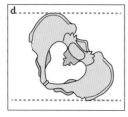

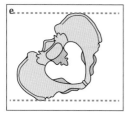

When researching the reliability of visual assessment of the lumbar spine, Fedorak et al (2003) asked therapists to assess whether lumbar spines were normal or whether there was increased or decreased lordosis. They found fair intrarater reliability but poor inter-rater reliability. It is therefore important for you to always make your own assessment of a client's lumbar posture and especially if you believe lumbar posture may be a contributing factor to symptoms and intend to perform postural assessment regularly in order to check progress.

It is important to note that changes in posture do not necessarily correlate to pain or to changes in pain. For example, Franklin and Conner-Kerr (1998) found that although lumbar lordosis and sagittal pelvic tilt increased from the first to the third trimester of pregnancy, these changes were not related to back pain.

Tip 3: A Trick for Identifying Pelvic Position

When assessing a client who is significantly overweight, it can be difficult to determine the position of the pelvis from postural assessment alone. Palpation is usually necessary in order to locate the anterior superior iliac spines (ASIS) for example. However, not all clients feel comfortable with palpation and, again, palpating through adipose tissue in order to determine pelvic position in standing can be difficult. The following "trick" can help determine whether your subject is standing with their pelvis in a neutral (a), anterior (b), or posterior (c) pelvic position.

1. In standing, begin by demonstrating to your client how to perform a posterior pelvic tilt and, if necessary, help reposition their pelvis into a posterior position when they are resting supine (see Chapter 7, Tip 1 for information on how to do this).
2. Next, demonstrate an anterior pelvic tilt (again in standing position).
3. Once you are certain that your client understands how to change the position of their pelvis, ask them whether it feels easier to move into an anterior pelvic tilt or into a posterior pelvic tilt position.

If a client finds it difficult to move into one of the pelvic positions, that could be because they are *already* in that position.

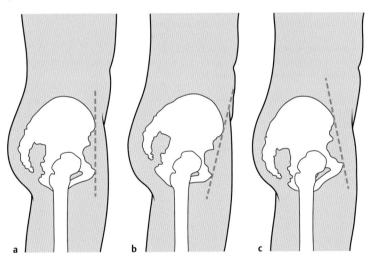

a　　　　　　　　b　　　　　　　　c

A client:
- Who finds it easier to move into an anterior pelvic tilt position is likely to be more posteriorly tilted.
- Who finds it easier to move into a posterior pelvic tilt position is likely to be more anteriorly tilted.
- Who can move easily between an anterior and a posterior pelvic tilt position could have a neutrally positioned pelvis.

Tip 4: Assessing the Effect of Sitting Posture on the Lumbar Spine

Backs dislike being retained in static postures, so when working with a client who sits for prolonged periods of time, it is useful to observe *how* they sit:

- At work.
- At home.
- When relaxing.
- When commuting.

Observing the sitting posture your client adopts when they sit is useful because it provides information as to the position the spine and pelvis are in for prolonged periods. Once you have this information, you can easily work out which muscles are shortened and which are lengthened and therefore the kinds of exercises that are necessary to alleviate pain that may result from fatigue in soft tissues. Sometimes a client deliberately adopts a posture they find alleviates their back pain, and this is also useful to know. Sometimes they can sit for prolonged periods on one type of chair but not on another, and may not know what it is about chairs that makes the difference. Minor changes in the height and tilt of the chair seat can have profound effects on symptoms because they change the posture of the lumbar spine.

TIP: One thing to remember is that when sitting upright:

- *Increasing* hip flexion tends to *decrease* the lumbar curve.
- *Decreasing* hip flexion tends to *increase* the lumbar curve. (Note this is not the case when a subject sits with a slumped posture, knees extended.)

The chart which follows details the posture of the lumbar spine that corresponds with different sitting positions. Remember to observe prolonged recreational postures too. For example, rowing, drawing, writing, gaming, and watching television.

For information about how seated postures alter lumbar spine apophyseal joints and intervertebral disk shape and function, please see Adams and Hutton (1985).

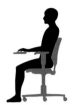

The lumbar spine retains its natural curve in normal, upright sitting with hips and knees at approximately 90 degrees.

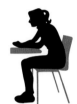

Leaning forward to rest the arms on a desk produces flexion at the hip and spine, reducing the lordotic curve.

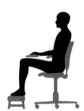

Sitting upright and using a footstool produces flexion at the hip and spine, reducing the lordotic curve.

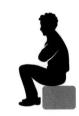

Sitting on a low chair produces flexion at the hip and spine, reducing the lordotic curve.

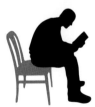

Resting the arms on the knees as when reading produces flexion at the hip and spine, reducing the lordotic curve.

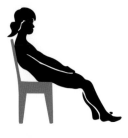

When slumped with knees extended, the pelvis tilts posteriorly and lumbar curve reduces.

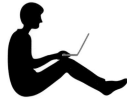

Sitting on the floor with a book or laptop as shown procures flexion of the hip and spine and reduces the lordotic curve.

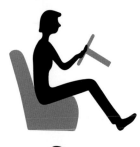

Leaning forward to drive results in either a neutral or a flexed lumbar spine depending on the degree of hip flexion: the greater the hips are flexed, the greater the degree of lumbar flexion.

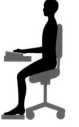

Tilting a seat downward at the front produces an anterior pelvic tilt and an increase in lumbar lordosis.

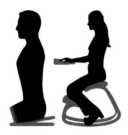

Using a wedge-shaped cushion to sit on tilts the pelvis anteriorly and produces an increase in the lumbar curve.

Using a "kneeling" chair or stool decreases hip flexion, tilts the pelvis anteriorly, and facilitates a more normal lumbar lordosis.

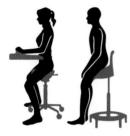

Using a "saddle" seat or "perch" stool reduces hip flexion, tilts the pelvis anteriorly, and facilitates a more normal lordotic curve.

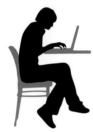

Sitting with the legs crossed or sitting on a thick wallet raises the pelvis on one side and produces lateral flexion in the lumbar spine.

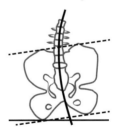

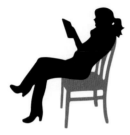

Combinations of postures are also possible. For example, sitting in a slumped posture with the legs crossed produces posterior pelvic tilt and both rotation and lateral flexion of the lumbar spine.

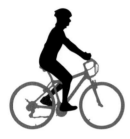

Cycling posture varies: when upright, the spine is in a more neutral position, although not likely to retain the normal lumbar curve; when bending toward the handlebars as when using a racing bike, the lumbar spine is flexed.

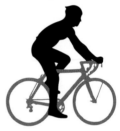

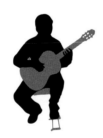

Using a footstool on one leg as is common when playing classical guitar produces increased hip flexion on the footstool side, raises the pelvis, and, therefore, laterally flexes and forward flexes the spine.

As you can see, different ways of sitting affect the lumbar curve. Remember also that sitting and standing affect the spine differently. When assessing patients with low back pain, Lord et al (1997) found that lumbar lordosis in standing was on average 50% greater than lumbar lordosis in sitting. So if your client spends a lot of time standing, their standing posture may be more significant than their seated posture. Although there is little evidence to support a relationship between pain and posture, this may be more to do with the types of questions that have been asked and the assessment that was done, and there may in fact be a relationship between posture and pain (Sahrmann 2002).

Tip 5: **Sleeping Positions**

When working with clients with lumbar pain or stiffness, it is useful to enquire how they sleep. Information about your client's sleeping position may help you to do the following:

- Identify whether the position is aggravating an existing condition.
- Determine the likelihood of a lumbar problem occurring in asymptomatic clients.
- Determine the cause of an existing problem—clients often adopt the posture opposite to that which causes the problem. For example, if flexion produces pain relief, the problem could be with extension of the lumbar spine.

You can then use this information to help plan your treatment and advise your client.

The following table describes the position of the lumbar spine in some common sleeping positions.

Sleeping position	Lumbar spine position
On stomach 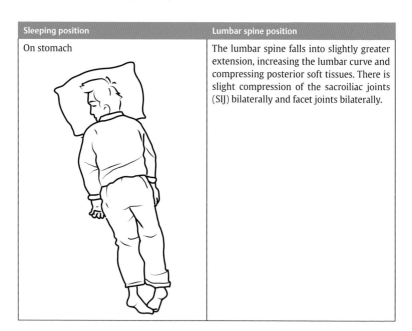	The lumbar spine falls into slightly greater extension, increasing the lumbar curve and compressing posterior soft tissues. There is slight compression of the sacroiliac joints (SIJ) bilaterally and facet joints bilaterally.

On back	The normal lumbar curve begins to decrease as gravity pulls the vertebrae toward the mattress as muscles relax. However, this may not be the case in clients with tight iliopsoas because with the hips in neutral, psoas may pull lumbar vertebrae anteriorly, temporarily increasing the lumbar lordosis.
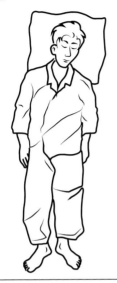	
On stomach with one hip flexed	Flexion of the hip produces a slight decrease in lumbar lordosis. The pelvis is raised on the side the hip is flexed with lateral flexion of the spine (concave on the side of hip flexion) and rotation of lumbar vertebrae. Facet joints are compressed on the side of hip flexion. Depending on whether a pillow is placed beneath the flexed knee, there may be slight gapping of the SIJ on the flexed hip side (reduced with use of a pillow) and compression of the SIJ on the opposite side. Overall, the pelvis is torsioned: the side of the neutral hip is in neutral or anterior pelvic tilt, while the side of the flexed hip is in posterior pelvic tilt.
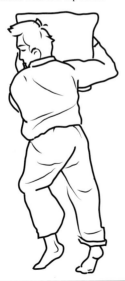	

Sleeping position	Lumbar spine position
On back with knees flexed 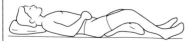	The lumbar curve is decreased because hip flexion in this manner produces a posterior pelvic tilt and slight flexion of the lumbar spine.
On side with hips and knees flexed, knees touching 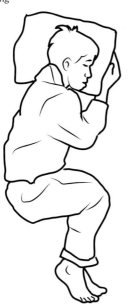	The lumbar curve is decreased because hip flexion produces a posterior pelvic tilt and slight flexion of the lumbar spine. The greater the degree of hip flexion, the "flatter" the curve of the lumbar spine becomes. There may be slight "gapping" of the SIJ and lengthening of posterior lumbar tissues to a greater extent than when resting supine with the knees flexed. 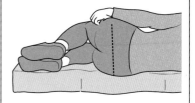
On side with one uppermost knee falling toward mattress 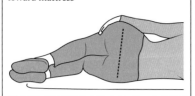	The lumbar curve is decreased due to the posterior pelvic tilt induced by hip flexion. There may be slight rotation of the lumbar spine as the pelvis rotates to follow the direction of the uppermost limb. There is slight compression of the facet joins on the side of the spine closest to the mattress.

Tip 6: Assessing Lumbar Range of Movement

As with the neck and the thorax, when a client comes to you with symptoms affecting their low back, it is helpful to assess the range of movement (ROM) that they have in their lumbar spine. Hypermobility or hypomobility in the lumbar spine could be contributing to symptoms locally or in the lower limbs or both. You may well have come across a client who hurt their back and then experienced symptoms in their legs. Sciatica is a common example.

It is difficult to isolate ROM to the lumbar spine when performing these tests because movements in lumbar spine segments are always accompanied by movements of the thorax:

- Lumbar rotation is accompanied by lateral flexion of the thorax to the opposite side.
- Lumbar lateral flexion is accompanied by thoracic rotation to the opposite side.

Lumbar and Thoracic Movements

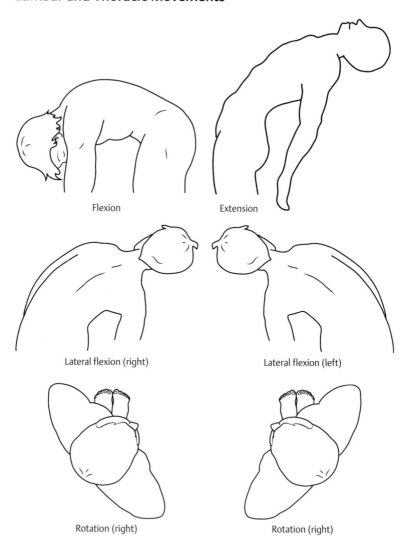

Flexion

Extension

Lateral flexion (right)

Lateral flexion (left)

Rotation (right)

Rotation (right)

One of the best ways to assess ROM in the lumbar spine is to perform the movements yourself, one at a time, and then ask your client to try and perform the same movement. Observe not only the range through which your client can move, but also how they move.

Ask yourself the following questions for each movement that is performed:

- Is the movement fluid or is it jarring?
- Does the client appear to be in discomfort?
- Does the client use compensatory movements to achieve the one you are asking them to perform?
- Are they willing or hesitant to perform the movement?
- Are you able to discern at this stage what might be hindering a movement? For example, fear? Spasm? Pain? Anatomical restriction?

TIP: During the subjective section of your assessment, you are likely to have gained some ideas as to the sorts of movements that may bring on your client's symptoms. Therefore, it is advisable to ask your client to perform those movements last. If you are new to assessing clients in this way, you may find Tip 7 useful as it provides a chart showing which movements of the lumbar spine are associated with a selection of daily activities.

TIP: If, during the subjective assessment, your client reports that a particular movement aggravates their symptoms, yet when performed with you this same movement does not bring on any symptoms, it is sometimes worth asking your client to maintain the position for 15 seconds.

ROMs are highly variable between different segments of the lumbar spine and also between different age groups: ROM decreases as we age.

	Normal lumbar ROM[a]
Flexion	40 degrees
Extension	30 degrees
Lateral flexion	20–30 degrees
Rotation	10 degrees

Abbreviation: ROM, range of movement.
[a] Data from Kapandji (2008)

Some Advice on Checking Lumbar Rotation

There are various ways to observe lumbar rotation. Two of the most common ways is with your client standing or seated.

In standing position, your client can move their hips and legs, and in so doing may appear to have a greater degree of rotation than when the hips are stable. It could be argued that ROM assessment with your client seated is a more accurate method because the pelvis is stabilized.

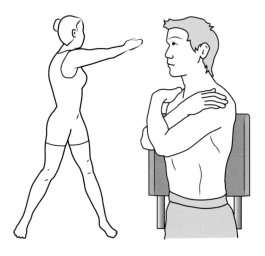

TIP: Whether you observe the client standing or seated, avoid looking at their head. Focus your attention instead on their torso and ask yourself how far they have managed to rotate their torso from their pelvis.

Use the following chart to experiment with the difference between standing lumbar rotation and seated lumbar rotation. Assess three subjects, asking each to rotate to one side as far as they can first in standing and second in seated position. Document your observations.

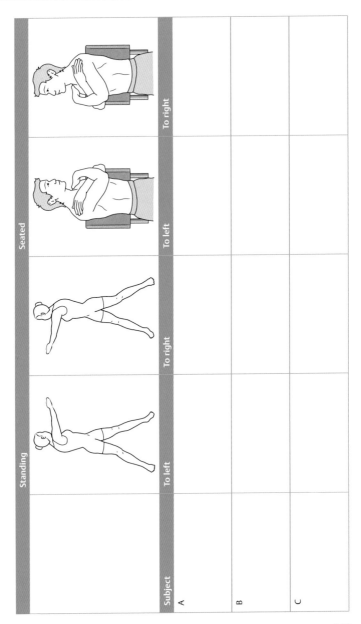

Subject	Standing				Seated			
		To left	To right			To left	To right	
A								
B								
C								

Tip 7: Lumbar Range of Movement during Daily Activities

Often, a client will report that they cannot identify what brings on their back pain. However, with questioning they sometimes remember that, after performing a particular activity, their pain was worsened. This is helpful to you as a therapist because you can identify what movement or combination of movements may have occurred in their spine during that activity. Physiotherapists, osteopaths, and chiropractors train in order to be able to reproduce these combined movements passively, usually adding slight overpressure to determine if symptoms are replicable. However, this book is aimed primarily for massage therapists and you may not have had this training and may not be insured to assess clients in this manner. Nevertheless, you could still provide advice on the avoidance of activities that either already aggravate or could aggravate your client's symptoms.

The following table provides examples of daily activities and the lumbar movement associated with each. If, for example, your client reports they start to get symptoms when leaning over to brush their teeth, you can see from the table that this involves flexion and so activities which involve flexion should be temporarily avoided.

Daily activity	Range of movement required[a]
Brushing teeth	Mild forward flexion.
Washing up	Mild forward flexion.
Using a broom	Mild forward flexion.
Lifting a refuse sack out of a dustbin	Medium forward flexion when leaning to grasp the sack, then loaded extension to lift the sack out of the bin itself.
Vacuuming	Mild-medium forward flexion.
Bathing a child	Forward flexion.
Putting on socks or footwear	Full forward flexion.
Loading a low-level washing machine	Flexion.
Unloading a low washing machine and lifting basket of washing	Flexion followed by extension with considerable compression.
Hanging washing	Extension when pegging/unpegging washing; flexion to retrieve wet washing if the basket of washing is low.
Using an oven	If the oven is low, flexion and extension accompanied by loading of the spine if holding something heavy such as joint of meat or casserole.
Gardening	Varies: bending forward to hoe or weed or bed-in plants involves flexion; reaching to one side to get plants while kneeling adds rotation; lifting peat, for example, involves loaded extension, often from a flexed position; digging involves flexion and rotation with considerable compression into extension.
Sitting up straight	Extension.
Turning around in seat to reverse a vehicle	Rotation.
Lifting shopping into/out of a car boot	Flexion + extension + rotation.
Getting into a car	Flexion + rotation.
Getting out of a car	Rotation + flexion.
Washing windows, dusting high shelves	Extension + rotation + lateral flexion.
Reaching up to pull a curtain closed	Extension + rotation + lateral flexion.

[a]Note that most daily activities involve a whole range of combined movements and people have different ways of doing things. If a subject has low back pain, they may also have developed a movement strategy that is not "normal" in order to lessen the likelihood of pain. Sometimes this is done consciously and sometimes unconsciously.

Tip 8: Locating Quadratus Lumborum

Much has been written about quadratus lumborum (QL), and therapists are often encouraged to treat this muscle manually. However, in order to treat it with hands-on techniques, it is necessary to locate it with palpation. Muscle charts often show muscles in isolation (as in the one on the right) and while this can be helpful in showing muscle attachments, it is easy to forget how deep this muscle lies in the body.

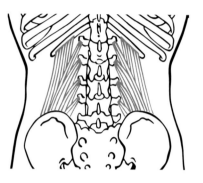

Observe the cross section of the lumbar region shown in the following illustration. Notice how QL lies deep to the erector spinae group and to two layers of fascia, the posterior and middle thoracolumbar fasciae that house the erector spinae.

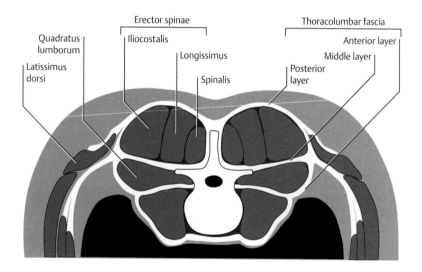

To locate QL, position your subject prone and stand to one side of the couch. Place your hands on their waist on the opposite side to you. That is, if you are standing on their left side, reach over to their right-side waist. With firm pressure, gently drag your fingers through the soft tissues. The first "block" that you feel is QL and almost immediately you also meet the erector spinae group.

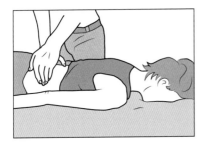

One way to be sure you have located the muscle is to ask your client to "hitch" their hip on that side. QL is (among other things) a hip hitcher and therefore will contract when they perform this movement, and you will feel the contraction.

Question: Why can't I just get my client to laterally flex or extend their spine in order to palpate this muscle?

Hitching up the hip on one side (a) is easier than trying to laterally flex the body (b) when in the prone position. Also, when attempting to laterally flex, or when performing extension (both movements brought about by QL), the erector spinae also will contract, so you could not be sure whether you had identified QL or the erector spinae.

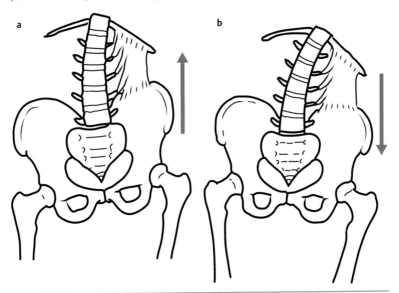

Tip 9: Appreciating the Function of Erector Spinae

As therapists, we are taught how everything is interconnected and how one body part affects another. You can perform a very simple test to remind yourself about the significance head movements have to the lumbar spine. You can use the erector spinae muscles to demonstrate this. (The test can later be used to help educate your client about the effect of the head on their lumbar spine, and particularly about the importance of head posture).

1. Position your client prone, their face downward. Use a face cradle or hole in the massage couch if possible.

2. Place your fingers on the erector spinae either side of the spine in the lumbar region, just below the waist, and press firmly but gently. It is important that you palpate while your client is relaxed and not speaking.

3. Maintaining your pressure, ask your client to lift their head and turn it to one side. What do you notice? As soon as they lift their head, the lumbar erector spinae contract. This is because the entire spinalis group (and associated fascia) contracts in order to lift the head from the couch and support it while it is being turned to one side.

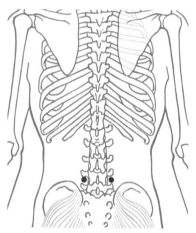

Take home message: Lifting the head against gravity has a significant effect on the lumbar erector spinae. Movements of the head also affect the lumbar spine in the upright position as when sitting or standing, but to a lesser degree.

TIP: There is an easy way for English-speaking therapists to remember the positions of the erector spinae muscles which all run vertically down the spine.

Stand behind your subject. From the outside (lateral) to the inside (medial), run your fingers three times vertically down the back and with the first movement say "I" (1), with the second movement say "love" (2), and with the third movement say "standing" (3). ("I Love Standing.") Your hand movements correspond with the names of the erector spinae muscles, that is:

I = iliocostalis.
Love = longissimus spinalis.
Standing = spinalis.

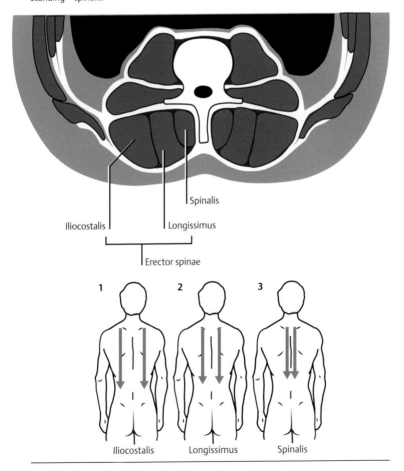

Tip 10: Quebec Back Pain Disability Questionnaire

In addition to observation, ROM, muscles length tests, and palpation, it is also sometimes helpful to use a specific test for the assessment of pain or disability. The Quebec Back Pain Disability Scale (QBPDS) is one such test and is in the form of a questionnaire (Kopec et al 1996).

This is a questionnaire used to measure functional disability of clients with low back pain. It contains a list of 20 daily activities that the client ranks according to the level of difficulty: not difficult at all, minimally difficult, somewhat difficult, fairly difficult, very difficult, or unable to perform at all. Answers can be collected using this Likert-type scale. That is, from 0 = no effort to 5 = unable to. The higher the score, the greater the level of functional difficulty.

You will find the questionnaire listed below. Following it, you will find examples of two completed questionnaires. In the first example, the client's questionnaire is scored at 37 corresponding to a low-level back pain that does not affect their daily function. The second questionnaire is scored at 74, indicating a much higher level of disability. (Note, numbers 0–5 and column totals have been added to the examples so you can better see how the score was calculated.)

Disability questionnaire	Not difficult at all	Minimally difficult	Somewhat difficult	Fairly difficult	Very difficult	Unable to
1 Get out of bed	☐	☐	☐	☐	☐	☐
2 Sleep through the night	☐	☐	☐	☐	☐	☐
3 Turn over in bed	☐	☐	☐	☐	☐	☐
4 Ride in a car	☐	☐	☐	☐	☐	☐
5 Stand up for 20–30 min	☐	☐	☐	☐	☐	☐
6 Sit in a chair for several hours	☐	☐	☐	☐	☐	☐
7 Climb one flight of stairs	☐	☐	☐	☐	☐	☐
8 Walk a few blocks (300–400 m)	☐	☐	☐	☐	☐	☐
9 Walk several miles	☐	☐	☐	☐	☐	☐
10 Reach up to high shelves	☐	☐	☐	☐	☐	☐
11 Throw a ball	☐	☐	☐	☐	☐	☐
12 Run one block (about 100 m)	☐	☐	☐	☐	☐	☐
13 Take food out of the refrigerator	☐	☐	☐	☐	☐	☐
14 Make your bed	☐	☐	☐	☐	☐	☐
15 Put on socks (pantyhose)	☐	☐	☐	☐	☐	☐
16 Bend over to clean the bathtub	☐	☐	☐	☐	☐	☐
17 Move a chair	☐	☐	☐	☐	☐	☐
18 Pull or push heavy doors	☐	☐	☐	☐	☐	☐
19 Carry two bags of groceries	☐	☐	☐	☐	☐	☐
20 Lift and carry a heavy suitcase	☐	☐	☐	☐	☐	☐

Kopec, J.M., Abrahamowicz, M., Abenhaim, L., Wood-Dauphinee, S., Lamping, D.L. and Williams, J.I. 1996. The Quebec Back Pain Disability Scale: conceptualization and development. J Clin Epidemiol. Feb;49(2):151-61.

As a client improves, whether as a result of
your treatment or from some other means,
their overall score should go down.

Example 1	Not difficult at all	Minimally difficult	Somewhat difficult	Fairly difficult	Very difficult	Unable to
	0	1	2	3	4	5
1 Get out of bed	☒	☐	☐	☐	☐	☐
2 Sleep through the night	☐	☒	☐	☐	☐	☐
3 Turn over in bed	☒	☐	☐	☐	☐	☐
4 Ride in a car	☐	☒	☐	☐	☐	☐
5 Stand up for 20–30 min	☐	☐	☒	☐	☐	☐
6 Sit in a chair for several hours	☐	☐	☒	☐	☐	☐
7 Climb one flight of stairs	☐	☒	☐	☐	☐	☐
8 Walk a few blocks (300–400 m)	☐	☒	☐	☐	☐	☐
9 Walk several miles	☐	☐	☒	☐	☐	☐
10 Reach up to high shelves	☐	☐	☒	☐	☐	☐
11 Throw a ball	☐	☐	☒	☐	☐	☐
12 Run one block (about 100 m)	☐	☐	☐	☒	☐	☐
13 Take food out of the refrigerator	☐	☒	☐	☐	☐	☐
14 Make your bed	☐	☐	☒	☐	☐	☐
15 Put on socks (pantyhose)	☐	☐	☒	☐	☐	☐
16 Bend over to clean the bathtub	☐	☐	☐	☒	☐	☐
17 Move a chair	☐	☐	☐	☒	☐	☐
18 Pull or push heavy doors	☐	☐	☐	☒	☐	☐
19 Carry two bags of groceries	☐	☐	☐	☒	☐	☐
20 Lift and carry a heavy suitcase	☐	☐	☐	☒	☐	☐
	0	5	14	18	0	0
	Total = 37					

Example 2	Not difficult at all	Minimally difficult	Somewhat difficult	Fairly difficult	Very difficult	Unable to
		1	2	3	4	5
1 Get out of bed	☐	☐	☐	☒	☐	☐
2 Sleep through the night	☐	☐	☐	☐	☐	☒
3 Turn over in bed	☐	☐	☐	☒	☐	☐
4 Ride in a car	☐	☐	☒	☐	☐	☐
5 Stand up for 20–30 min	☐	☐	☐	☒	☐	☐
6 Sit in a chair for several hours	☐	☐	☐	☐	☐	☒
7 Climb one flight of stairs	☐	☐	☒	☐	☐	☐
8 Walk a few blocks (300–400 m)	☐	☐	☒	☐	☐	☐
9 Walk several miles	☐	☐	☐	☐	☒	☐
10 Reach up to high shelves	☐	☐	☒	☐	☐	☐
11 Throw a ball	☐	☐	☐	☐	☒	☐
12 Run one block (about 100 m)	☐	☐	☐	☐	☐	☒
13 Take food out of the refrigerator	☐	☐	☒	☐	☐	☐
14 Make your bed	☐	☐	☐	☐	☒	☐
15 Put on socks (pantyhose)	☐	☐	☐	☐	☒	☐
16 Bend over to clean the bathtub	☐	☐	☐	☐	☐	☒
17 Move a chair	☐	☐	☐	☐	☐	☒
18 Pull or push heavy doors	☐	☐	☐	☐	☒	☐
19 Carry two bags of groceries	☐	☐	☐	☐	☐	☒
20 Lift and carry a heavy suitcase	☐	☐	☐	☐	☐	☒
	0	0	10	9	20	35
	Total = 74					

Tip 11: Relevance of Hip Flexor Length to Lumbar Assessment

Hip flexor muscles affect the lumbar spine because they have the ability to pull the pelvis anteriorly. This creates an increase in the normal lumbar curve, increasing lordosis in that region of the spine. If this is not countered by hip extensor strength, the im- balance could contribute to discomfort and pain in the low back. There are several dif- ferent ways to test the length of hip flexor muscles. Two examples are the prone knee bend test and the Thomas test.

Prone Knee Bend Test

With your client in the prone position, flexion of the knee tests the length of knee extensors, including rectus femoris, which crosses the hip anteriorly. Holding the an- kle, observe your client's lumbar spine as you passively flex their knee. Where rectus femoris is particularly tight, you will notice that the lumbar spine moves—there is a very slight increase in anterior tilt. Spinous processes of lumbar vertebrae move closer together and soft tissue of the low back are compressed. Note that very little movement in the spine is required to aggravate low back pain, and some clients with a short- ened rectus femoris muscle may feel not only a stretch down the front of their thigh, but also discomfort in the low back. Move- ment in the lumbar spine occurs because rectus femoris is being passively lengthened and so pulls on the anterior inferior iliac spine, from where it originates. Knowing that rectus femoris may be shortened is use- ful because lengthening it may help reduce anterior tilt and therefore reduce symptoms in the low back in some cases.

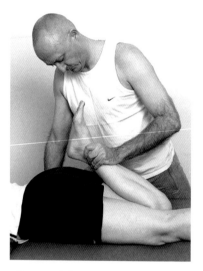

For more information on these tests, see Kendall et al (1993).

Thomas Test

The Thomas test, named after Hugh Owen Thomas, a British orthopaedic surgeon, is used to assess for shortness in hip flexor muscles. Position your client supine on the edge of a treatment couch. Take care that the couch will not tip up—plinths are heavy and stable, but massage tables are not. As your client leans backward, ask them to hold one leg but to avoid pulling it in too tightly toward their chest. Doing this gives a false impression of hip flexor tightness on the opposite hip, the one you are testing. In this position, the hip should be able to rest flat on the treatment couch, or even drop down slightly below this. (It is for this reason that it is important your subject is on the edge of the couch because if the thigh rests on the couch, you cannot tell whether there would have been greater hip extension if the couch surface were not in the way.) The following illustrations indicate some possible findings:

a. Slightly less than normal hip flexor length
b. Shortened rectus femoris
c. Shortened hip flexors

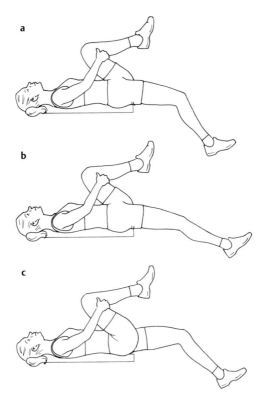

Tip 12: Measuring Lumbar Range of Movement Using a Tape Measure

One method of measuring ROM in the lumbar spine is with skin distraction. Two standard points of measurement are marked on the skin overlying the spinous processes of the lumbar spine and then the distance between these is measured when the subject flexes or extends. During flexion, the marks move further apart; during extension, they move closer together. The two points of reference you will need to identify are L1 and the start of the sacrum (S1).

STEP 1 Locate L1 and S1 on your subject. Measure the distance between these two points and record your findings.

STEP 2 Ask your client to flex. Measure the distance and record your findings.

STEP 3 Starting in a neutral position again, ask your client to extend. Measure the distance and record your findings.

In Standing

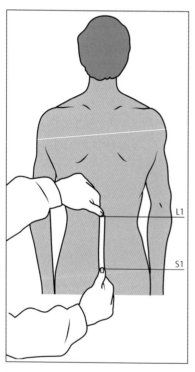

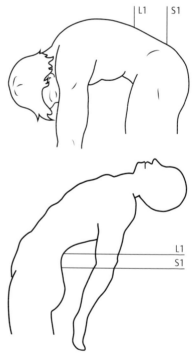

Note that you are likely to get different results depending on whether your client is standing or sitting. It is nevertheless useful to be able to take measurements in both positions because you may have a subject who cannot stand due to lower limb injury, for example. Conversely, you may have a client who finds sitting uncomfortable, due to coccygeal pain.

Use the following table to compare your findings when measuring a subject in standing and sitting positions. Practice on five subjects and record your findings in the table on the following page.

In Sitting

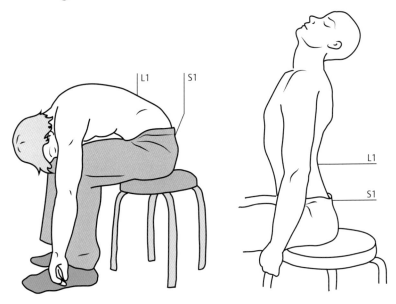

	Neutral L1–S1	Flexion	Extension
Standing			
Sitting			

Subject	Neutral L1–S1	Flexion	Extension
A			
B			
C			
D			
E			

Tip 13: Normal Lumbar Spine Range of Movement

Measuring lumbar ROM in clinical practice is difficult. The following illustrations show the lumbar ROM of middle-aged subjects measured using radiographs. These figures are taken from the American Academy of Orthopaedic Surgeons (Greene and Heckman 1994) and are based on three studies: Dvorák et al (1991) and Pearcy et al (1984a, b, two studies). If you have taken measurements with your subjects seated, you may observe a difference between these figures and your own findings because data here is for subjects in the standing position. (Full lumbar flexion cannot be achieved in the sitting position.)

Flexion/extension 70–7.69 degrees.

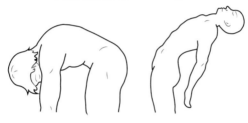

lateral flexion (right to left) 40–49.8 degrees

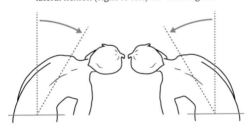

rotation (right to left) 12 degrees

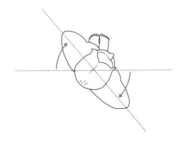

Chapter VIII

Lumbar Treatment

Chapter 8 **Lumbar Treatment**

There are fewer treatment tips in this chapter than in other chapters. The reason is that those that are provided here cover important aspects of lumbar spine treatment that are often neglected, and which require greater explanation. They include tips such as how to really facilitate a posterior pelvic tilt (and why), how to overcome spasm in lumbar muscles, and methods to traction the lumbar spine safely. An exercise to reduce the effects of a mild scoliosis, which I have termed "Klapp's creeping crawl," is included as a super example of thinking outside of the box, as the saying goes. We really do need to start to think in different ways about the treatment of the lumbar spine, not just in the techniques we use, but also in the contribution we can make as therapists over and above the delivery of hands-on treatments. The crawling exercise has not been validated, nor has the reliability of the technique been established. Yet it demonstrates how someone many years ago (around 1904) was brave enough to propose an exercise that may have seemed strange but for which there was a sound rational.

The tip on treating clients with back pain is another example of how we as therapists can put our advanced knowledge to good use to help inform our clients. It can be all too easy to forget that the knowledge we gain while training and through years of experience that subsequently follow is not familiar to the majority of our clients, despite the enhanced availability of health information in today's society. Treatment for symptoms in the low back can certainly be hands-on, but more than ever, providing support in the form of education about the management of back pain, or the prevention of symptoms occurring in the first place, is paramount.

Tip 1: Trick to Facilitate a Posterior Pelvic Tilt

The ideal pelvic posture is for the pelvis to rest in a neutral position (a) with the anterior superior iliac spines (ASIS) on the same vertical plane as the pubis. In this position, the lumbar spine rests with a slight curve, concave posteriorly.

However, some people have an increased lumbar curve (hyperlordosis), and this can cause pain due to compression of soft tissue structures posteriorly. Being able to actively reposition the pelvis from an anterior pelvic tilt position (b) in which the ASIS fall anterior to the pubis, to a posterior pelvic tilt position (c) in which the ASIS fall posterior to the pubis is useful for three reasons:

- The movement itself serves as a form of mobilization, increasing mobility in this region of the spine and reducing stiffness.
- In order to bring about the movement, it is necessary to contract the abdominals, something which can be done in either standing or supine positions and which is a safe abdominal strengthening exercise, even for people with lumbar problems.
- Once in the posterior position (c), the lumbar extensor muscles begin to relax and the overlying fascia is stretched slightly, sometimes reducing discomfort.

Unfortunately, many clients do not know what the posterior pelvic tilt position feels like and therefore struggle to bring this about. One way you can facilitate this is to manually move the pelvis for your client. Some osteopaths and chiropractors place their hands on the sacrum and move the pelvis manually, but this could be considered inappropriate when performed by a massage therapist. A less intrusive method is to use a towel.

1. With your client in the supine position, hip and knees flexed, ask them to help position a towel beneath their back. The most effective position is for the towel to begin at the base of the thorax, high up on the lumbar spine.

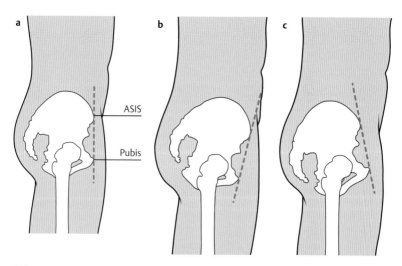

2. Still with hips and knees flexed, feet on the couch, encourage your client to relax. (You do not want them to lift their bottom off the couch as if performing a bridging exercise.)

3. Using a series of short tugs, tug the towel from beneath your client. In doing so, you will gently tug on the pelvis, repositioning it so that it rests in the posterior tilt position. Ask your client for feedback: they should report that their back feels more straight and some may report now being able to feel the couch with their back, which they were unable to feel before.

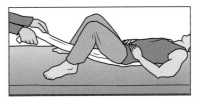

Question: Why can't I just pull the towel out from the client? Why do I need to tug it out?

The tugging method seems to produce a greater posterior tilt position, but you could experiment with towel removal and select the method that works best for you.

TIP: Some clients may wish to hold their trousers if these are loose, as the trousers sometimes get pulled down at the back by the towel.

Tip 2: Using a Towel to Passively Relax and Stretch the Lumbar Spine

Gentle rocking can have a relaxing, sedative effect and reduce tone in muscles. Using a towel to rock the body in the tip described here is one way to facilitate this.

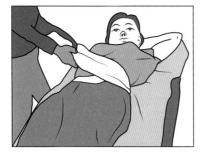

1. Fold a towel such that its width approximately matches the size of the space between your client's iliac crest and their rib cage.
2. Next, lay the towel across your couch and help your client to get comfortable in the supine position with the towel positioned behind their waist.
3. Standing to one side of the couch, take up the end of the towel on the opposite side from you. Holding this end of the towel, very gently pull the towel towards you and notice that it gently lifts one side of your client's waist from the couch.

Use this technique to apply a gentle, rhythmic motion and thus "rock" your client on one side before repeating the technique on the other side of the body.

TIP: Notice that if your client reaches one arm above their head, this facilitates a stretch on that side of the body.

Question: For how long should I "rock" the body like this and during which part of the treatment?

You do not want to make your client feel seasick by rocking too vigorously—too frequently or with too much force—the idea is to relax, not stimulate. Most clients cannot feel that there is a towel placed horizontally beneath their waist if you position it here at the start of the treatment, so you can make use of the technique whenever it feels appropriate.

Tip 3: Minimizing Lumbar Disk Pressure

In 1970, Swedish researchers Nachemson and Elfström published data they had obtained from inserting pressure needles into the L3 disk of different subjects and recorded the change in disk pressure when their subjects performed movements associated with everyday activities (walking, jumping, standing, and carrying, for example). Results (see bar chart on the following page) revealed that some activities considerably increased disk pressure.

Where there is an underlying problem, increased pressure can result in pain and neurological symptoms such as sciatica. Therefore, it is helpful to share this information with clients and encourage them to avoid activities likely to increase pressure on lumbar disks.

"Lifting wrong" is used to mean lifting with knees extended, bending at the waist, not keeping the load close to body.

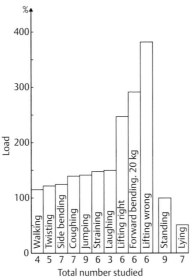

Based on Nachemson, A. and G. Elfström. 1970. Intravital dynamic pressure measurements in lumbar discs. Scand J Rehabil Med 2. suppl 1: 1-40.

Question: Which clients would benefit most from this information?

When a person suffers back pain, they do not need anyone to tell them that moving in a certain way will aggravate their pain; they know that leaning forward to put on their shoes, for example, is impossible, or that the jolt from a sudden cough exacerbates their pain. These kinds of clients tend to self-manage their symptoms by avoiding postures that worsen their pain. Clients who are currently pain free but who experience frequent reoccurrences have usually also learnt how to manage episodes of pain and can often tell when they have "overdone things," a "niggling pain" being the precursor to more debilitating symptoms. The kinds of clients who may benefit most from your advice are those who may only have experienced one episode of pain, which may be attributable to compression of a lumbar disk or facet joint, or overstretching of a lumbar ligament, and who have not yet experienced a reoccurrence. These clients may be unaware that some everyday activities are potentially harmful.

Nachemson and Elfström found that in a simple standing posture (A) pressure increased significantly when their subjects stood holding a 10-kg weight in each hand (B) and increased further still when they attempted to lift these weights with bent legs (C) and with straight legs (D).

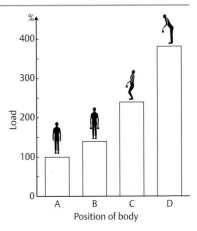

Tip 4: Avoiding Potentially Harmful Abdominal Exercises

Many clients report wanting to lose weight and to tone their abdominal muscles. It is popularly believed that increasing tone in abdominal muscles contributes to core stability and that core stability lessens the chances of experiencing back pain. While the exercises shown here are probably safe for healthy athletes, they place considerable pressure on disks of the lumbar spine and should therefore be avoided by people with a history of back problems or those who are currently in pain.

You learnt in Tip 3 that researchers Nachemson and Elfström measured interdiskal pressure in the lumbar spine during everyday activities. In the same study, they also measured pressures when subjects performed exercises that were commonly used at that time (1970) to strengthen abdominals. Findings revealed that in all exercises, disk pressure rose considerably. These findings indicate that these exercises are likely to be unsafe for subjects with lumbar problems and are not suitable for early-stage rehabilitation.

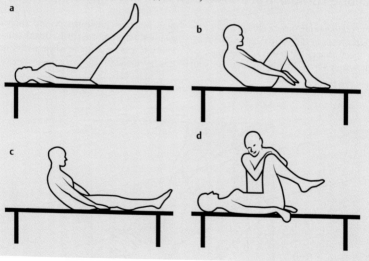

Nachemson and Elfström found that in bilateral straight-leg raising (a), lumbar disk pressure rose approximately 50% compared to standing, and by 100% in both flexed-knee (b) and extended-knee (c) sit-ups. When performing isometric abdominal contraction in the crook-lying position (d), pressure increased approximately 40%.

Tip 5: Five Ways to Traction the Lumbar Spine in Supine

Tractioning is useful for reducing spasm in lumbar muscles: separating vertebrae reduces pressure on neural tissues and may therefore be helpful in treating radicular symptoms in conditions such as sciatica. Described here are five methods of tractioning, each with a subtly different effect. Each method is performed with your client in the supine position and a chart has been provided at the end of this tip so that you can record your findings when practicing each method.

Question: Are there any contraindications to these techniques?

Yes. They should not be used on hypermobile clients or during pregnancy. Care is needed when using them within 12 months following pregnancy when ligaments may still be lax. Lower limb tractioning should be avoided if your client has a problem affecting their hip, knee, or ankle, or if holding the foot as described would be problematic. None of these techniques would be used to treat an acute injury. You should be certain that the cause of the back pain is muscle spasm, rather than another pathology. The methods described here are specifically for the purposes of reducing spasm in lumbar muscles.

Gentle Lumbar Traction Stretch with Sheet/Towel

Tractioning using this method provides a direct stretch to the lumbar spine. Wrapping a sheet around the pelvis of your client as shown in the illustration below, use your body weight as you lean backward, applying gentle traction to the pelvis. Guard against injury to your own spine when performing this technique.

TIP: You may find that this stretch is best applied with your client resting on a mat on the floor rather than on a massage couch.

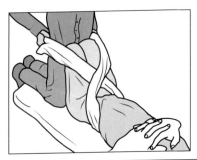

Gentle Lumbar Traction Stretch with Seat Belt

An alternative is to use a seat belt as a stretching aid. With your client in the supine position, hips and knees flexed and feet resting on the couch, place a looped seat belt around your own hips, at about buttock level. Then place the other end of the loop over your client's knees so that it rests on their upper thighs, a towel between their thighs and the belt. Once in place, all you need to do is to lean back gently, using your body weight to apply the traction.

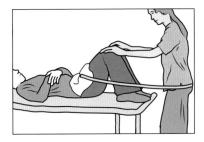

Gentle Gravity-Assisted Lumbar Traction Stretch

This stretch is best performed with your client on the floor, their hips and knees flexed as in the previous stretch. Providing they have no issues affecting their lower limbs, place your thigh beneath the legs of your subject and use it to support the weight of their lower limbs as you gently use the strength in your own limb to raise your client's hips off the floor and in so doing, provide gentle traction to the lumbar spine. If you are much shorter in stature than your client, then this stretch may not work. An alternative is to use a gym ball.

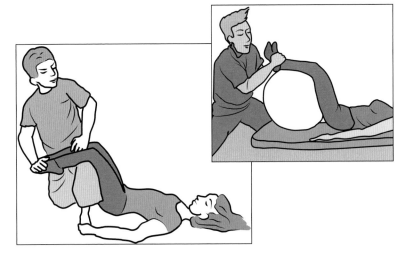

Gentle Unilateral Lower Limb Traction Stretch

This indirect stretch produces a very mild stretch in the lumbar spine on the side to which the traction is applied. Holding the ankle of one leg as shown in the illustration below, apply gentle traction by leaning backward.

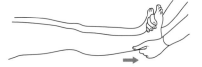

Gentle Bilateral Lower Limb Traction Stretch

This is also an indirect stretch and produces a mild stretch to the lumbar region as a whole. Place your client's legs together and with one hand cupping each heel, slowly lean back. It is difficult to exert much traction when holding both legs in this manner, which is why the stretch is mild.

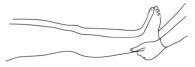

An alternative handhold, and one which produces slightly greater traction, is to place a towel horizontally beneath the ankles (a) and then to wrap it around the ankles, crossing it over the dorsum of the feet (b) as your client rests supine on the couch. Then, hold the ends of the towel (instead of the ankles) when leaning backward.

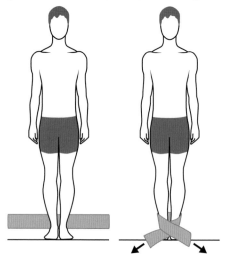

Technique	My findings
Lumbar traction using a towel	
Lumbar traction using a seat belt	
Gravity-assisted lumbar stretch	
Unilateral lower limb traction	
Bilateral lower limb traction (hands)	
Bilateral lower limb traction (towel)	

TIP: When performing traction using the leg techniques, you can achieve a greater reduction in muscle tone in the lumbar spine if you ask your client to perform a posterior pelvic tilt once you have applied the traction. This maneuver requires contraction of abdominals, the muscles opposing the erector spinae, and contraction of the opposing muscle reduces tone in the spasming muscles.

Question: Can you traction the lumbar spine in any other position?

Yes, in the side-lying position you can use the unilateral lower limb technique, applying it to the uppermost leg. Tractioning in the prone position is less effective, however, because in the prone position the lumbar spine adopts its normal, if not slightly exaggerated, lumbar curve. This places muscles in a shortened position where they are more likely to cramp again. On the other hand, in the supine positions described in this tip, the lumbar spine flexes slightly, reducing the lumbar curve, ever so slightly lengthening soft tissues, and therefore facilitating a reduction in tone.

Tip 6: Treating Spasm in Lumbar Muscles

Sometimes, acute pain experienced by a client in their lumbar region is due to spasming of muscles. Spasm is an involuntary, usually temporary, contraction in the muscle. In the lumbar region, it is revealed as a palpable increase in tone, often in the erector spinae muscles and is frequently unilateral. Sudden spasm resolves of its own accord within a short period of time, but when prolonged, treatment is useful in providing relief from pain.

Some of the techniques described here are easier to apply than others. They do not need to be applied in any particular order and you may find that you only need to use one technique to reduce the spasm and symptoms.

Supine Lower Limb Rocking

This technique mimics that of a passive "chi" machine, a device that gently sways the client's legs from side to side while they rest supine. Cupping your client's ankles in your hands, gently sway these side to side in a swinging movement. There is no need to lift the legs far from the table, just enough to facilitate the movement. Obviously, if your client has heavy legs, you may choose not to apply this technique. The side-to-side movement does not need to be of large amplitude to be effective. What seems to be effective is the rhythmic back-and-forth rocking that begins to relax tissues of the lumbar spine and in doing so reduces muscle spasm.

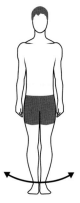

Be careful of your own posture when performing this technique and guard your own back, as you are supporting the weight of both of your client's limbs. It is fatiguing to perform this movement for more than a few minutes, but it could be interspersed with other techniques you intend to use in the supine position.

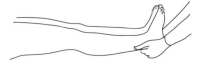

As you perform this technique, think about how it is affecting the longitudinal muscles of the spine. Before moving your client's legs, their pelvis is level and the spinal extensor muscles are parallel (a). If you move the legs to one side, the pelvis tilts, and there is slight compression of soft tissues on the side you are moving to but slight lengthening of the tissues on the side you are moving away from (b).

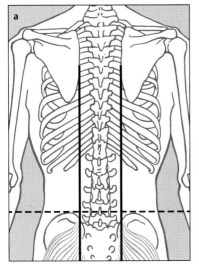 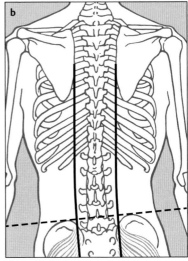

TIP: Leaning back slightly while swaying the client's legs gently tractions and therefore simultaneously stretches the tissues of the back, albeit only slightly. In some cases, this could provide enough relief and rocking may not be necessary.

Supine Stretch and Rocking

Stretching reduces muscle tone. To passively stretch the lumbar extensors with your client in the supine position, flex their hips and knees and gently push these knees toward the chest, increasing the degree of hip flexion.

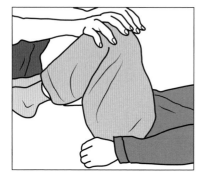

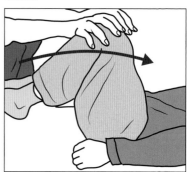

If your client is comfortable, apply gentle overpressure (i.e., increasing hip flexion further) once in the fully flexed hip position. This produces a posterior pelvic tilt and lengthening of lumbar extensor muscle and fascia.

This stretch may not be possible when treating clients with pendulous abdomens or hip flexor pain. It should not be used in clients with replacement hips on one or both sides.

Facilitated Posterior Pelvic Tilt Stretch

If the supine stretch and rocking technique is not possible, you could position your client similarly, with hips at 90-degree flexion, and then ask your client to perform a posterior pelvic tilt. (For information on how to teach this posterior pelvic tilting, please see Tip 1.) Performing a posterior pelvic tilt requires contraction of abdominal muscles and doing so reduces tone in the spasming muscles of the lumbar spine.

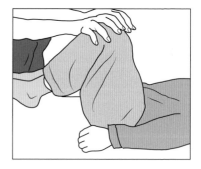

Static Pressure

In the prone position, lengthen the tissues of the lumbar spine by placing a pillow beneath your client's stomach (a). Apply gentle static pressure to the lumbar muscle that is spasming (b). It is likely to be one of the erector spinae muscles running vertically on one side of the spine. Maintain your pressure for about 60 seconds, during which time your client should experience a reduction in symptoms. Repeat up to five times on other parts of the muscle.

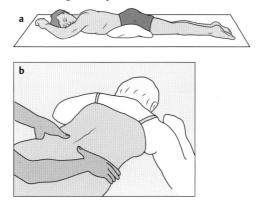

Static Pressure and Stretch in Fetal Position

This technique can be quite difficult to apply but is nevertheless useful. With your client resting in a fetal position, apply gentle pressure to the spasming muscle. Maintaining this pressure, ask your client to either flex further at the waist or perform a posterior pelvic tilt. Either of these movements lengthens the lumbar erector spinae muscles and helps to stretch them while you are also applying static pressure. Notice that in the following illustration the therapist has chosen to stand at the head of the client, but you can also stand behind the client if you prefer. Take care with your own posture when performing this technique, and avoid overstretching your own spine.

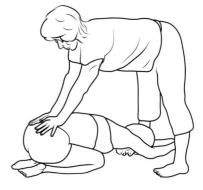

Static Pressure and Stretch in Sitting Position

An alternative is to perform the technique with your client sitting on the couch, and you standing behind them. The disadvantage of the sitting position is that there is a tendency to push the client forward, and for them to resist this. In doing so, they contract their erector spinae, the very muscles you are trying to relax. Once you have applied pressure to the spasming muscle, ask your client to "slump" or to perform a posterior pelvic tilt, both of which will lengthen the lumbar extensor muscles. Avoid using your thumbs if your thumb joints are hypermobile or sore.

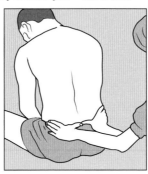

Isometric or Concentric Contraction of the Opposing Muscle Group

Contraction of the opposing muscle is a common method for reducing tone in a spasming muscle. However, it can be challenging to use this method when treating erector spinae. Contraction of the abdominals occurs during the posterior pelvic tilt maneuver, and this could be all that is required to reduce the spasm. An alternative is to attempt a sit-up, lifting the head and shoulders just a few inches off the floor (a and b), a movement that requires stronger contraction of the abdominals. You would need to be certain that the effort of performing the sit-up is not counterproductive. That is, the increase in global muscle tone brought about by a deconditioned subject when attempting to perform a sit-up does not aggravate their lumbar spasm.

a
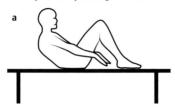

b
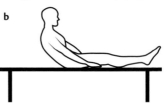

Positional Release Technique

Positional release is another technique used to reduce tone in spasming muscles. In this technique, the muscle is taken into an even shorter position than it is presently in. Attempting to use positional release technique in the lumbar spine is tricky because most people have difficulty shortening the muscles of the lumbar spine comfortably, as this necessitates additional extension of the spine.

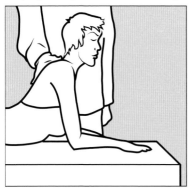
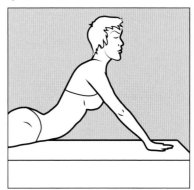

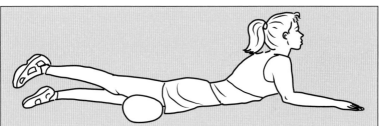

One method is for the client to rest in the prone position and to push themselves up onto their elbows. For positional release technique to work, it is necessary for the client to relax as fully as possible, with the affected muscle shortened in the position of least pain. Therefore, you could facilitate this by placing a pillow beneath the thighs, still in the prone position, so both the hip and spine are taken slightly into extension.

Traction

This gently stretches the muscle. For examples and details of how to apply traction, please see Tip 5.

Prone Rocking

Another way to use rocking is to position your client prone, and, standing to one side of the couch, place your hand on the side of their pelvis and gently "rock" this away from you. In so doing you bring about a slight rotatory stretch in tissues as the low thoracic spine remains still and the lumbar spine is gently rotated due to the movement of the pelvis. This technique is described in full in Tip 13.

Massage

Massage can be useful in reducing muscle tone. Use a pillow beneath the stomach to reduce the lumbar lordosis and slightly lengthen the tissues of the lumbar spine. Broad, slow, and firm strokes used over a wide area are likely to reduce tone, whereas light, fast, strokes to a specific area are likely to increase tone.

Advice on Avoidance

If your client is prone to lumbar spasm, it would be useful to assess postures they adopt on a daily basis. Muscles are prone to cramp when they are kept in shortened positions. Therefore, it is important to know whether your client adopts postures that require prolonged lumbar extension, lateral flexion, rotation, or any combination of these. Common examples of positions that may require shortening of lumbar muscles are as follows:

- Not sitting squarely in front or a computer monitor (rotation).
- Sitting with one leg crossed over the other (lateral flexion).
- Leaning back (as when painting a ceiling) (extension).
- Leaning back and twisting like when placing the hand over the passenger seat in a vehicle in order to twist the body to look through the rear window (rotation and extension).

Summary of Techniques to Reduce Muscle Spasm

Technique	Comments
Supine lower limb rocking	
Supine stretch and rocking	
Facilitated posterior pelvic tilt stretch	
Static pressure	
Static pressure and stretch in fetal position	
Static pressure and stretch in sitting position	
Isometric or concentric contraction of the opposing muscle group	
Positional release technique	
Traction	
Prone rocking	
Massage	
Postural observation and advice	

Question: Are there any disadvantages to reducing muscle spasm in the lumbar region?

Yes. Muscles may spasm to protect an underlying problem. Good examples are where there has been a facet joint injury such as impaction of the joint or lesion in an associated ligament or where there has been a lumbar herniation. In such cases, reduction in the hypertonicity of the affected muscles provides pain relief of only the most temporary nature: as soon as your subject attempts to move, the spasm reoccurs. One way to think of this type of spasm is as a form of splinting, just as one might splint a fracture: the erector spine of the lumbar region may go into spasm to reduce movement in a lumbar segment when there has been an injury.

Tip 7: Klapp's Creeping Crawl

You may have observed that some clients have a slight lateral curvature to their lumbar spines, and in cases of scoliosis this could be quite pronounced. One of the challenges of scoliosis is that there is reduced strength in lumbar extensor muscles, and this could have consequences for participation in sports and may affect daily activities.

Orthopaedic surgeon Rudolf Klapp developed a series of exercises that involved asymmetrical stretching postures and strengthening exercises. These were based on his observations of quadrupeds that do not develop scoliosis. Crawling on all fours was known as Klapp's "creeping" exercise and although it was later abandoned for use by children because they developed knee problems, it is still worth reconsidering for use with adults.

Iunes et al (2010) photographed 16 subjects with idiopathic scoliosis before and after treatment using these exercises and concluded that the Klapp method was an efficient therapeutic technique for treating asymmetries in the trunk.

It is not clear how many exercises need to be performed or how frequently. Iunes et al used 20 treatment sessions for their study.

Although a wide variety of exercises was used by Klapp, consider the simple crawl movement. There are few clients for whom this would be unsafe, the only disadvantage being pressure through the knee and possibly the upper limb. For that reason, it should not be used by clients with knee problems or arthritis in the upper limb. Consider two variations on the crawling movement and try these for yourself.

Simple Straightforward Crawl on Hands and Knees

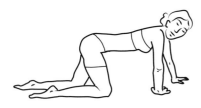

In order to perform this movement, the spine is required to laterally flex side to side to correspond with the tilting movement of the pelvis as each leg is brought forward in turn, yet without the weight of the upper body. The effect is to mobilize the lumbar spine symmetrically.

If you practice this for yourself, you may notice that your waist is slightly compressed on the side that you bring one knee and leg forward, due to elevation of the pelvis on that side, but not to a very great degree. Although this is an unorthodox method of treatment by today's standards, it is useful to reexamine corrective exercises such as the one put forward by Klapp.

Simple Straightforward Low Crawl on Elbows and Knees

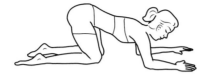

A variation is to perform the crawl with the weight supported more through the forearms, a position which is supposed to require less muscular effort and greater elongation of tissues.

You may discover if you practice this for yourself that it is uncomfortable on the neck as the posterior neck muscles work to extend the neck as the head is held against gravity. Keeping the neck in alignment with the spine—that is, with the face towards the floor rather than raised—reduces this discomfort.

Crawling to Correct a Lumbar Curve

Klapp argued that by crawling around in a circle, with the convexity of the curve on the inner side of the circle and the concavity on the outer side, muscles on the inner side would be required to contract within their inner range and the purpose is to reduce the curve. For example, if you had a client with a laterally curved lumbar spine that was convex on the left and concave on the right, you would encourage them to crawl around in a circle anticlockwise.

For left-sided convexity and right-sided concavity

For right-sided convexity and left-sided convexity

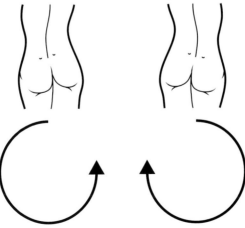

Use the following table to practice these four techniques and notice how your spine feels with each.

Technique	Comments
"Walking" on hands and knees in straight line	
"Walking" on elbows and knees in straight line	
"Walking" on hands and knees in a circle	
"Walking" on elbows and knees in a circle	

Tip 8: Treating Clients with Back Pain

The most effective treatment therapists can provide is not with hands-on techniques; it is with the information they impart. One group for whom this is particularly helpful are those clients suffering from back pain.

Not surprisingly, many clients with back pain are fearful, anxious, frustrated, and sometimes become low in mood. Often, they have many unanswered questions.

Question: What sorts of questions might be asked by a subject with back pain?

- Why have I got back pain?
- What is causing my pain?
- Why have I not got a diagnosis?
- What if the diagnosis is bad news?
- What if I have a serious back problem?
- Why is my pain persisting?
- How long will it last?
- What if it won't go away?
- Is there anything I can do to stop this happening again?

This tip provides ideas as to the kinds of information likely to reassure a client with acute back pain. The focus of this tip is on explanation, reassurance, and education regarding self-treatment:

- *Explanation* regarding causes of back pain.
- *Reassurance* that most back pain is not an indication of serious injury.
- *Education* encouraging the client to take control of their pain and start moving sooner rather than later.

The information provided in this tip has been split into manageable sections. You could use it to create your own list of bullet points. Such a list could be given to clients for whom you felt it was appropriate or you could simply use it as an aide–mémoire when treating clients with back pain.

As there is so much information about treatment for back pain, only general information has been provided here. You will find specific information about exercises and coping with daily life in Chapter 9.

Causes of Back Pain

Using a picture or an anatomical model is helpful when describing the structures thought to be responsible for back pain.

- The spine is made up of bones (vertebrae) and bones can cause back pain, but this is extremely rare. (Bone pain could result from a fracture or bone cancer. Compared to all of the other causes of back pain, cancer is the least common, and it is important to stress to your clients that back pain due to cancer is extremely rare. However, it may be unwise to go into this level of detail when providing information to clients who could become fearful on hearing the word "cancer.")

- Bones are held together by ligaments. Ligaments are tough tissues that can be wrenched. Wrenching of a ligament is known as a sprain. You could reassure your client that the ligaments of the back can be sprained just like ligaments of the ankle. You might further reassure them that while sprains are extremely painful, they are not serious.
- The spine contains facet joints. These are small joints where part of one vertebra joins another vertebra. Jarring or jamming a facet joint is painful as this pushes the joint surfaces together. Again, this is painful but not serious.
- Between the body of each vertebra is a disk of cartilage. This is extremely strong. In some cases, cartilage herniates and the popular term for this is a "slipped disk." Cartilaginous disks do not actually "slip." They are like toffees and can squash out to one side between bones. This causes extreme pain when the bit of the disk that squashes out presses on a nerve. Often there is leg pain if the nerve goes down the leg. Usually when the disk returns to a more normal position, any leg symptoms resolve.
- Very strong muscles support the back, along with tough tissue called fascia. Both muscles and fascia can be torn. Again, this is painful but not serious.
- Sometimes back pain is worsened by feelings of anxiety and depression. The structures involved may not be particularly damaged, but the subject's fear and anxiety combine to produce sensations of extreme pain. Explain to your client that reducing their anxiety can reduce their symptoms.
- There are some forms of back pain for which the cause is unknown.

Diagnosing Back Pain

- Back pain can therefore originate from a variety of anatomical structures, and could even be the result of minor injury to more than one structure at the same time (such as a ligament and a muscle). This makes diagnosis difficult.
- X-rays and scans sometimes reveal serious pathology, but X-rays are not particularly helpful for identifying minor injury, even when this is painful. Most back pain is the result of minor injury or is termed "mechanical" low back pain, meaning it is related to the mechanics of the back rather than a serious pathology.
- X-rays and scans sometimes reveal degeneration. Degeneration is normal and simply refers to the everyday wear and tear of joints that affects us all. Studies show that subjects with spines that are shown to be highly degenerated on X-ray do not necessarily have pain and that some subjects with a lot of pain do not appear to have degenerative spines. Therefore, having an X-ray that shows degeneration does *not* mean that the degeneration is the cause of the pain.
- It is frustrating, but we have to accept that in many cases we cannot identify the cause of pain.

Reassurance

- Most back pain is not serious. It may certainly be very painful, but that does not mean there is serious damage.
- Back problems are common. Many other people are likely to have experienced back pain of this kind.
- Many people experience a recurrence of their back pain. However, this can vary from many months apart to many years apart.
- Acute pain usually only lasts a few days.
- Where pain is the result of injury, normal healing processes take place. For a detailed description of the process of healing and repair, you might wish to read the article by Professor Tim Watson called "Soft tissue repair and healing review" (http://www.electrotherapy.org/assets/Downloads/tissue%20repair%202014%20Final.pdf). His article describes the complex process of events that take place during the healing process and gives an indication of the kinds of time span each process takes, noting that there is much overlap between phases and differences between individuals.

Treatment

It is important to explain to clients that how the medical profession treats back pain has changed. In the past, people were advised to rest. We now know that resting for more than about 1 to 2 days is not usually helpful and may worsen pain and lead to more disability. The focus now is on what the client does for themselves. This is because outcomes are known to be more favorable when a subject takes control of their pain rather than relying on the medical profession to "fix" them.

Question: Why is bed rest no longer recommended for people with back pain?

Resting in bed for more than a few days has a detrimental effect on the body and delays recovery.
- Bones weaken.
- Joints stiffen.
- Muscles weaken.
- Physical fitness declines.
- Depression is common.
- Pain usually worsens.
- The need for pain medication usually increases.

It becomes more and more difficult to get back to a normal way of living.

Examples of the sorts of advice you can give include the following:
- By all means lie down, but only when pain is so bad it limits you completely from doing any form of daily activity.
- You do not need pain to settle completely before returning to normal activities. Muscles waste with immobility, which can lead to further pain.
- Within a few weeks, pain has usually reduced to such a level that you can get on with everyday activities, taking care as you do these.
- Backs love movement. The sooner you are able to move, the better.

Why is physical activity good for people with back pain?

Physical activity improves physical and emotional well-being and therefore aids recovery. With physical activity:

- Bones become stronger.
- Joints become more mobile.
- Muscles strengthen.
- There is an improvement in fitness.
- Natural painkillers are released into the bloodstream.
- It generally improves feelings of well-being.
- Action that you take can be more effective than any medication or treatment provided by a therapist, so it is important to take control, to choose to incorporate small amounts of gentle physical activity as soon as you can. Accept that you may feel pain and discomfort initially but that, gradually, this will lessen and you will recover more quickly than if you lie in bed.
- People who decide to get on with their life cope better with back pain than people who give in to their pain.

Question: What sorts of physical activity is safe for someone with back pain?

Gentle, nonimpact exercise can hasten recovery without damaging the back, for example, swimming, cycling, or walking.

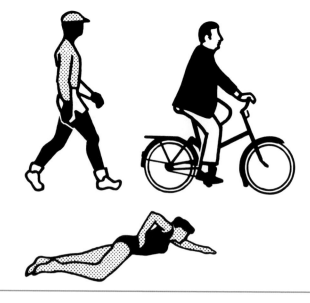

Tip 9: Taping the Lumbar Spine

Use of tape such as Kinesiotape (Kinesio Holding Corporation) has been postulated for use with clients with low back pain. As a relatively inexpensive and easy to perform application, there is a growing interest in research into this area of treatment. Applied over a lengthened muscle, the rationale for use of the tape is that it facilitates muscle function while permitting range of motion. This is believed to occur by stimulating the skin and, because the tape is elastic, elastic recoil of the tape itself. Another theory is that, because the tape is applied with the muscle in a lengthened position, and skin stretched, the convolutions that appear in the tape when the muscle is in a neutral position "lift" the skin and stimulate flow of superficial blood and lymph. Studies into the claims made by manufacturers are ongoing.

For example, a study by Lemos et al (2014) found that application of longitudinally placed parallel strips of tape increased forward flexion in healthy young women. A systematic review of four randomized controlled trials (Vanti et al 2015) concluded that there were too few studies on the effectiveness of the use of tape to draw any final conclusions.

This author has found that, using the longitudinal strips method, results are highly variable between subjects but that some clients with nonspecific low back pain report a reduction in low back pain after application of the tape and an increase in back pain on removal of the tape after about 3 days, but it cannot be certain whether this is due to the tape or placebo.

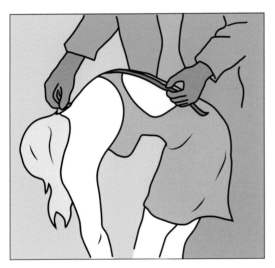
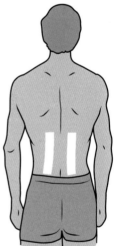

Tip 10: Stretching Hip Flexors

You learnt in this chapter that shortened hip flexors could pull the pelvis anteriorly, increasing the lumbar curve and contributing to low back pain. Stretching hip flexors could reduce this pull, help realign the pelvic to a more neutral position, and theoretically reduce back pain.

There are many ways to stretch hip flexors, and some of the simplest ways are shown in the following illustrations. Begin by testing the length of the hip flexors and record your findings. Apply the passive stretch for a minimum of 30 seconds and retest hip flexor length. Over time, reassess your client to see if this treatment has had any effect on their symptoms.

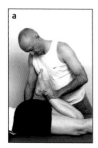
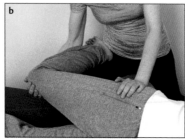

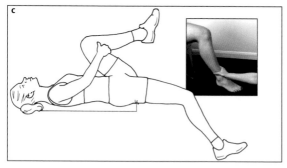

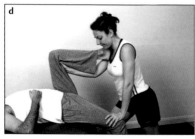

(a) Passive stretch to quadriceps, including hip flexor rectus femoris, in prone position. (b) Side-lying hip flexor stretch. (c) Supine stretch of rectus femoris. (d) Supine stretch of hip flexors.

Chapter IX

Lumbar Aftercare

Chapter 9 **Lumbar Aftercare**

As you may have come to discover by this part of the book, the tips that have been offered to you are based on my experiences of being a physical therapist and massage therapist for many years, working with the general population and those clients suffering in general with musculoskeletal conditions. One of the conclusions I have come to is that pain and stiffness in the lumbar region (but also in the neck and thorax) are exacerbated and may be caused by the retention of static postures for long periods of time. Therefore, the flavor of this aftercare chapter for the self-management of clients with low back complaints focuses on encouraging movement of the lumbar spine. Five of the tips are devoted to this topic alone and should provide you with enough ideas to be able to encourage any client with low back pain to move their back more often, in a variety of different positions, safely. Research supports and encourages self-management of symptoms for people with low back pain. This will never replace the soothing effects we can deliver with massage, nor the comfort of explaining a particular set of stretches, and there will always be a place for hands-on therapy in the treatment of patients with back pain. The aftercare tips provided here are designed to complement any existing treatments you have found to be effective and to provide you with another skill—that of being able to provide sound, supporting advice for the management of pain in the lumbar spine—to your clients.

Tip 1: **Bath Exercises**

Many people with back pain find relief from resting in a warm bath. Most are likely to lie still, fatigued from a day of lumbar pain and pleased to get some relief at last. You could use the information in this tip to educate such clients, explaining how simple movements, performed regularly, may be beneficial in reducing pain. The seven exercises described in this tip are designed to be performed in the bath and are indicated in the following situations:

- When it is not possible to treat a client because their low back condition is too acute.
- When your client is recovering from a period of immobility and their back feels stiff or where you have observed a reduced range of movement.
- When there is no further treatment, you can provide that will alleviate pain.
- In the early stages of rehabilitation following injury, providing the subject has medical approval.

The purpose of the exercises are to gently mobilize the lumbar spine, making use of the heated bath water for pain relief and the dimensions of the bath which purposefully limit the degree of movement that is possible.

Mobilization is likely to occur as a result of the following:

- A reduction in muscle spasm (if present) brought about by the water temperature.
- Gentle lengthening of lumbar muscles.
- Gentle movement of lumbar spine segments.

The exercises described here will have little effect on an asymptomatic subject but will enable a symptomatic subject to mobilize their lumbar spine safely, something they may be unable to do when not in the bath. All exercises are performed in the recumbent position and may be performed in any order. They are not intended to be performed vigorously, nor with any effort, and should be manageable. You could begin by suggesting that your client perform each one just a couple of times, for example.

Exercise 1: Partial Lumbar Extension

Place the hands in the water, palms touching the base of the bath. Keeping the legs outstretched, the buoyancy provided by the water enables a subject to lift their buttocks from the bath while still remaining submerged. Note that the object of this exercise is not to lift the hips out of the water, which could be potentially harmful, but only to lift the buttocks from the base of the bath, keeping the heels pressed to the base of the bath in order to bring this about. Very little effort is required from the hip extensors to perform this movement.

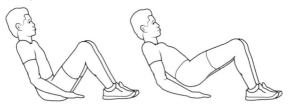

Effect: Partial lumbar extension produces very slight lumbar extension and may be useful for clients with a decreased lumbar curve. When combined with the posterior pelvic tilt, the effect is a gentle mobilization of the lumbar spine in an anterior–posterior direction.

Exercise 2: Posterior Pelvic Tilt

With the hands either in the water, palms touching the base of the bath, or resting comfortably on the sides of the bath, the client relaxes and, with the hips and knees comfortably flexed, uses their abdominals to bring about a posterior pelvic tilt.

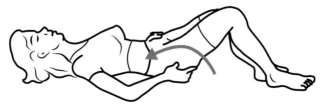

Clients unfamiliar with this pelvic movement will benefit from the advice provided in Tip 1 of Chapter 8 where you will find the description of a trick to help facilitate a posterior pelvic tilt. Soothed by the warmth of the water, when performed in the bath, this gentle exercise may be beneficial for clients with low back pain or those who report stiffness in this region.

Effect: Posterior pelvic tilt causes slight flexion of the lumbar spine, decreasing the lumbar curve, with lengthening of the lumbar extensors bilaterally.

Exercise 3: Unilateral Hip Flexion

With the hands either in the water, palms touching the base of the bath, or resting comfortably on the sides of the bath, the client simply flexes one hip and knee at a time, sliding the heel of one foot to the buttock on that side, and then slowly returns it to neutral.

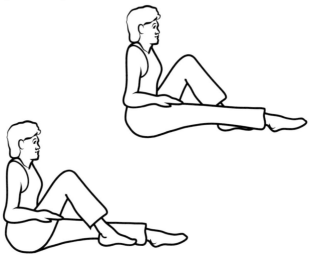

Effect: Unilateral hip flexion produces a mild posterior pelvic tilt, decreasing lumbar lordosis and lengthening lumbar extensors on the side of hip flexion.

Exercise 4: Bilateral Hip Flexion

This is usually easier with the hands in the water, palms touching the base of the bath but could be performed with the arms resting on the sides of the bath. Your client gently flexes both hips at the same time, sliding the heels toward the buttock, before returning them to neutral.

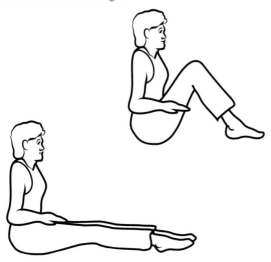

Effect: Bilateral hip flexion produces a mild posterior pelvic tilt, decreasing lumbar lordosis and lengthening lumbar extensors.

Exercise 5: Hip Hitching

Place the arms on the sides of the bath. The client "hitches" their right hip up, contracting quadratus lumborum (QL) by moving their right foot away from the end of the bath while keeping their leg straight. The client then attempts to "drop" the hip, attempting to touch the end of the bath with their toe, and does this several times before repeating on the left side.

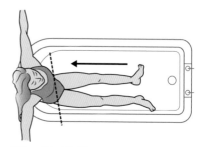

Effect: Hip hitching strengthens QL; hip "dropping" lengthens it; and it mobilizes the spine into lateral flexion.

Exercise 6: Leg Swaying

Place the arms on the sides of the bath. Keeping the legs outstretched and together, the client attempts to sway these from side to side, touching the lateral side of their right ankle to the right side of the bath, then swaying the legs together so that the lateral side of their left ankle touches the left side of the bath.

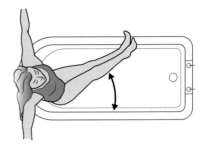

Effect: Leg swaying strengthens the muscles of lateral flexion both posteriorly and anteriorly and mobilizes the spine into lateral flexion.

Exercise 7: Partial Lumbar Rotation

Place the arms on the sides of the bath. One of the easiest exercises to perform in the bath, the client keeps their ankles together, hips and knees flexed, and simply lets their knees fall to the right and then to the left. The sides of the bath prevent full rotation. However, clients with shorter legs, or when the exercise is performed with the knee less flexed, achieve fuller rotation to each side.

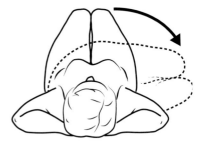

Effect: This exercise provides slight lengthening of lumbar muscles and mobilization of the lumbar spine into rotation.

TIP: Before giving these exercises to a client, practice them for yourself and make notes about how easy (or difficult) they are, and anything else that may help you give instructions to your client. Notice how the buoyancy of the water makes these exercises much easier than when they are usually performed "dry." Decide whether these may be suitable for your client.

Exercise	Comment
1. Partial lumbar extension	
2. Posterior pelvic tilt	
3. Unilateral hip flexion	
4. Bilateral hip flexion	
5. Hip hitching	
6. Leg swaying	
7. Partial lumbar rotation	

Tip 2: Self-Traction

Traction has been used for centuries as a treatment for back pain. Here are four safe and simple positions your client could use to self-traction their lumbar spine. Practice these yourself and decide whether one or more might be suitable for your client. Use the table ("My findings") provided at the end of this tip to make notes and to document any ideas you have for alternative items that could facilitate the position, plus any tips you want to be sure to give to your clients when attempting these positions.

How to Use Self-Tractioning Positions

- You might suggest that your client practice a different position for a few days and decide whether it reduces their symptoms. Clients are likely to have their own preferences. For example, a hanging traction may be more suitable to someone who lifts weights and wants to "decompress" their spine afterward.
- The most effective stretches are adopted for a period of about 30 seconds, and performed regularly. Whether your client can rest in any of the positions shown here for that length of time is likely to be variable.
- Position "A" may be used in an acute stage, providing it does not exacerbate symptoms.
- Each could be performed twice daily: once in the morning and once in the evening.
- The more relaxed your client feels, the more beneficial the traction is likely to be; therefore, traction positions "A" and "B," discussed in the following sections, are likely to be the most effective.

Position A

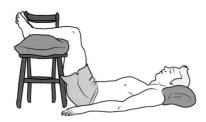

Experimentation is needed to get the height of the chair correct for this position, which should elevate the legs so that the hips "hang," thus tractioning the lumbar spine. Symptomatic subjects are likely to need assistance in positioning the chair or cushion to the correct height. A sofa, a bed, or a bench could be used equally well.

Position B

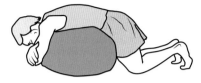

This subject is resting over a gym ball, but a small stool or pouffe could be used. In this example, the subject's knees are touching the floor. Ideally, the knees should not touch the floor at all because it is counterproductive to use the knees for support. The hips should "hang."

Position C

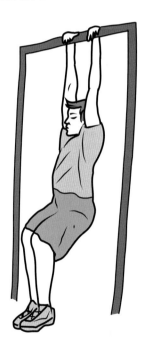

Here your client simply hangs, letting the weight of the hips and lower limb produce the traction. It requires good upper limb strength. Anything can be used from which to hang, providing it is strong and immovable, such as a tree branch, pull-up bar, or the horizontal bar of a goal frame. This tractions the upper limb and should not be used if your client has a history of subluxation or dislocation of the shoulders or elbows.

Position D

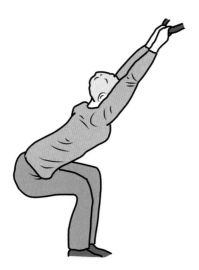 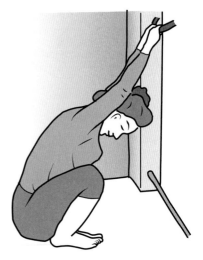

This is a similar but slightly different to position C. In position D, a strap is used to hang from and you can see that, because the body is not directly beneath the arms, the lower limb supports more of the weight and therefore tractions the lumbar spine less. (Practice positions C and D for yourself and you will see the difference.) However, anoth-er difference is that in position D, the hips are flexed to a greater extent, so the lumbar curve is reduced more than in position C as hip flexion produces a posterior pelvic tilt. As with position C, this tractions the upper limb and should not be used if your client has a history of subluxation or dislocation of shoulders or elbows.

My findings

Position	Notes, ideas, tips
A	
B	
C	
D	

It is not known how traction reduces symptoms, nor what dose is necessary for it to be effective. Several suggestions have been put forward for the mechanisms involved. For examples of these, please see Krause et al (2000). Sustained traction could be beneficial in acute cases of low back pain, but there is no evidence that traction reduces symptoms of nonspecific low back pain over and above other treatment methods (see Beurskens et al 1997, for discussion).

The ideas provided in this tip are simply that, ideas only. They are based on personal experience of working with clients with low back pain, originating from postural tension rather than disk compression or osteoarthritis. The rationale for their use is that they help lengthen and stretch soft tissue of the lumbar spine which may have become compressed due to immobility. Note that there are many studies of traction other than the two cited here.

Tip 3: Encouraging Movement of the Lumbar Spine – General Advice

People with pain in the lumbar region of the spine often seek help from people other than their doctor. This may be because they have been prescribed medication that no longer seems to be effective or because they do not wish to take analgesics. If you are reading this as a massage therapist, you may have been approached many times by clients hoping that massage will alleviate their symptoms. While massage can ease pain, musculoskeletal pain is often aggravated by the retention of a static posture—whether such posture is lying, sitting, or standing—and encouraging movement is a good thing. Part of our work as a therapist is to help clients find ways to self-manage symptoms on a daily basis. Not

surprisingly, however, people with back pain avoid movement, having found that initially this aggravated their symptoms or because they are scared, believing that moving might damage themselves further. As a consequence, people with low back pain often find themselves trapped in a cycle that perpetuates their pain:

1. They have back pain.
2. They avoid movement.
3. With inactivity, muscles weaken and joints stiffen, and sometimes muscles spasm. This leads to more pain (1). So the client avoids movement (2). And so it continues.

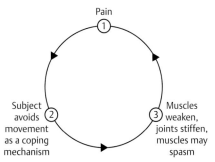

Pain
①

Subject avoids movement as a coping mechanism ②

Muscles ③ weaken, joints stiffen, muscles may spasm

In the majority of cases, with reduced movement pain is worsened over time, whereas with gentle movement pain is eased over time. We can play an important role in educating clients about this, offering them gentle encouragement and reassurance as they cautiously begin to move their

backs. You do not need to be a fitness expert or an exercise specialist to encourage clients with back pain to move more. The exercises shown here are safe and gentle. There are, of course, some clients for whom these would be contraindicated, and you can find information about those in the question box.

General Advice When Working with Clients about to Incorporate Gentle Back Movements into Their Daily Life

- It does not matter which exercise your client selects. They should start with the one they find easiest to perform.
- A good starting point is for the subject to perform each movement about three to five times.
- Performing the exercises daily is likely to bring about the most relief. These are mobilization exercises and are not the same as the kinds of exercises you might do in a gymnasium, where you need to give your muscles a day or two of rest in between.
- Movement could be uncomfortable but should not worsen pain or other symptoms such as sciatica.
- If symptoms do worsen, the exercise should be stopped.
- Performed daily, clients will often report an improvement in symptoms within 3 to 5 days. They should therefore be encouraged to persevere with the exercises unless these worsen symptoms.

- Keeping a diary is a useful way of recording which exercises have been performed, any improvements the client notices, as well as any challenges.

In the pages that follow, you will find a wide range of simple, safe exercises that may be performed in the side-lying, supine, kneeling, sitting, and standing positions. These have been separated into different tips because it is likely that your client may only be comfortable with one set of exercises and so you should focus on that group first. There is no ideal starting point: some clients find standing easier than lying, but you are equally likely to find clients for whom standing—or sitting—is intolerable. It is therefore important to enquire as to the kinds of positions your client prefers to rest in, in order to achieve a degree of relief, and to select exercises from the group that most closely matches that position.

Question: Are there any clients for whom these sorts of exercises are contraindicated?

Yes, these are not suitable for clients:

- Immediately postoperatively following surgery to the lumbar spine. Such exercises *are* often used as part of rehabilitation but when a subject is an inpatient and under the care of a rehabilitation team who follow a specific protocol.
- Following trauma such as a fracture to the lumbar region or pelvis where *immobility* is temporarily necessary to facilitate healing.
- Where there is an unhealed wound in the lumbar region.
- Where the low back pain is undiagnosed and may not be mechanical, e.g., in cases of vertebral tumor.

These exercises are often prescribed to patients following surgery or recovering from serious injury. If you are in any doubt as to whether they are appropriate for your client, then do not use them.

For an interesting review of disuse in chronic low back pain patients, please see Verbunt et al (2003). For recommendations regarding activity in patients with low back pain, articles such as that by Abenhaim et al (2000) are extremely helpful. We tend to think of acute low back pain as being highly disabling, requiring complete bed rest. However, some studies recommend activity. For example, Malmivaara et al (1995) concluded, "Among patients with acute low back pain, continuing ordinary activities within the limits permitted by the pain leads to more rapid recovery than either bed rest or back-mobilizing exercises" (p. 351).

Tip 4: Encouraging Movement of the Lumbar Spine – Side-Lying Techniques

The movements shown in this tip encourage flexion of the spine. Flexion of the spine may be brought about by actively curling the spine but also occurs when the hips are flexed. When performing the exercises, your client need not flex both hips/knees simultaneously.

Please read Tip 3 before using these techniques with your client.

A modification of this exercise is to flex only the top leg, then to change to resting on the other side of the body and flex the other leg. However, the process of changing from resting on one side to the other can itself be problematic and painful for many clients.

Exercise 1

Resting on whichever side is most comfortable, perhaps with a cushion between the thighs, knees, or ankles (a), the hips and knees are slowly flexed (b) as far as is comfortable and then returned to the start position (c).

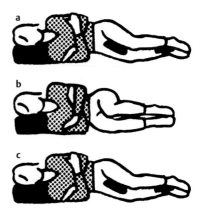

Exercise 2

An alternative is for the client to use their hands to gently draw the knees toward the chest, encouraging lumbar flexion (a). (Or the client could ease their torso toward the knees.) The aim is to bring about greater hip flexion and therefore an induction in the lumbar curve (b). In either case, the client returns to the starting position (c) following gentle flexion of the spine.

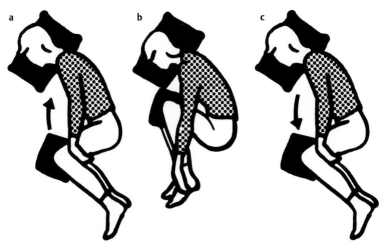

Exercise 3

If your client is anxious or unable to move their legs, they could remain in the side-lying position (a) while performing a posterior pelvic tilt (b). This is a flattening of the lumbar curve brought about by contracting the abdominals. You can find more information on the posterior pelvic tilt in Tips 1 and 2 in Chapter 8.

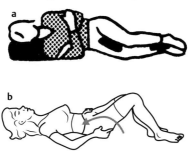

Tip 5: Encouraging Movement of the Lumbar Spine – Supine

In the supine position, the lumbar spine changes from a position of flexion to extension depending on the position of the pelvis. As the hip is flexed, the spine flexes; as the hip is returned to neutral, the lumbar spine extends slightly as it regains its normal lordosis. Straightening the legs in the supine position can be extremely uncomfortable for some clients; therefore, it is best to attempt to straighten only one leg at a time.

Please read Tip 3 before using these techniques with your client.

Exercise 1

Starting with the hips and knees gently flexed (a), your client slowly extends the knee of the right leg, straightening that leg (b). Once the leg has been straightened, it is returned to the start position (c) and the movement repeated using the left leg (d).

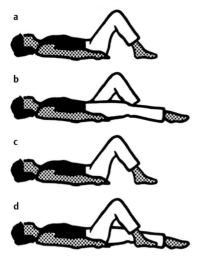

Exercise 2

Beginning with the hips and knees gently flexed (a), the right leg is gently brought closer to the chest (b), increasing flexion at the hip and lumbar spine. The leg is returned to the start position (c) and the exercise repeated on the left leg (d).

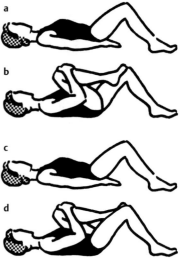

Exercise 3

Beginning with gentle hip and knee flexion (a), first one and then both hips and knees are flexed (b). In this position, the client moves their knees in a circular motion first clockwise (c) and then anticlockwise (d) before returning to the starting position.

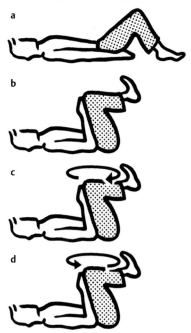

Exercise 4

With hips and knees gently flexed (a), the client flexes the right knee and holds it as they extend the left leg (b). Once in this position of right knee flexion and left knee extension, they let go of their leg and the arms are gently raised above the head so that they rest by the ears (c). Then the client returns to the start position (d). The movement is repeated on the other side.

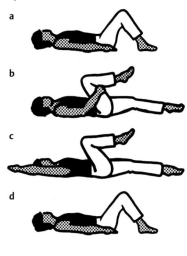

Exercise 5

This exercise encourages extension of the lumbar spine and may not be comfortable for all clients. With hips and knees gently flexed (a), the client slowly extends the right leg (b), then the left leg (c), and then raises the arms above the head so that they rest by the ears (d). The movement is then reversed: the arms are brought back to the side of the body, the left leg flexed, and finally the right leg flexed, bringing the client back to the start position.

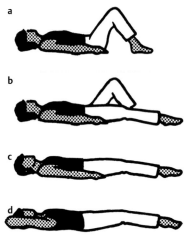

Exercise 6

If your client is reluctant to perform movements with their legs, they could simply practice increasing lumbar flexion by performing a posterior pelvic tilt. The client rests with hips and knees flexed and tries to flatten their lower back, pressing it toward the floor, using their abdominal muscles. For additional information, please see Tips 1 and 2.

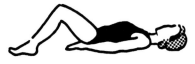

Exercise 7

Hip hitching is a movement often used to strengthen the lateral flexors of the spine, but it may also be utilized as a gentle mobilization exercise. It is usually performed with the knees extended, but this can be uncomfortable for some clients who may wish to attempt the movement with hips and knees flexed. The client "hitches" their hip up, contracting QL on the left (a) and then reverses the action, contracting QL on the right (b).

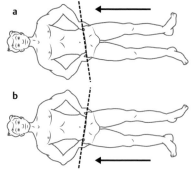

Tip 6: Encouraging Movement of the Lumbar Spine – Kneeling or Sitting

The exercises shown here involve very small movements of the lumbar spine and may be helpful for reducing pain and stiffness and in helping a client with back pain to return to normal activities. Exercises may be performed in any order, beginning with whichever your client finds most comfortable.

Please read Tip 3 before using these techniques with your client.

Obviously those exercises may not be suitable for clients who struggle to bear weight through their knees or upper limbs.

Exercise 1: Encouraging Flexion

In this very simple exercise the client begins in four-point kneeling (a) and then sits down onto the ankles (b), lowering the torso if possible. By doing this, the spine changes from a neutral position to one of slight flexion.

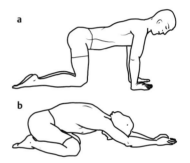

Exercise 2: Four-Point Kneeling Back Arch

Resting on all fours, the back is arched upward (a) and then downward (b), producing a flexion/extension movement in the lumbar spine.

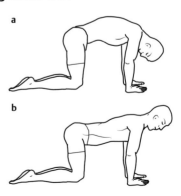

Exercise 3: "Walking" a circle

In four-point kneeling, imagine the knees are at the center of a circle and the hands are on the rim of the circle (a). "Walk" the hands to the right, as if moving them along the rim of the circle in that direction (b). The lumbar spine starts to flex laterally. The further the hands walk, the greater the degree of lateral flexion. Rotation is involved. A client needs to "walk" only a few inches, "walk" back, and repeat to the left.

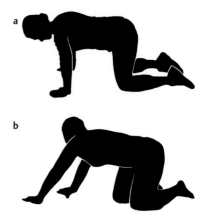

Exercise 4: Unilateral Hip Flexion

Begin on all fours (a). Transfer weight to the left knee. Slowly flex the right hip, bringing the right knee off the floor and bring it toward the chest (b). Return to the start position and repeat with the left leg. This creates a change from a neutral lumbar position to one of slight lumbar flexion.

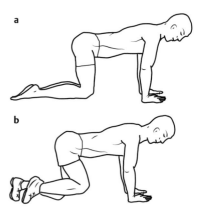

Exercise 5: Four-Point Kneeling Rotation

Resting on all fours (a), take the right arm and reach beneath the chest, trying to touch the floor to the left (b). In order to perform this movement, the spine rotates slightly. Repeat on the other side.

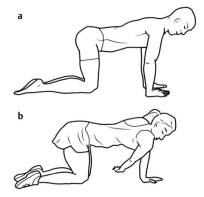

Exercise 6: Knee Marching in Sitting

From a sitting position, lift one knee from the chair and then return it. Repeat with the opposite knee. Alternate this gentle marching-type manner. The knee does not have to be lifted far from the chair. The higher the knee is lifted, the greater is the degree of lumbar flexion produced.

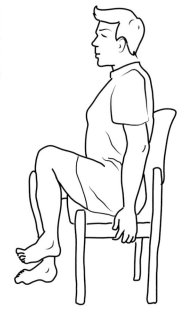

Exercise 7: Encouraging extension

To encourage extension of the lumbar spine, place the fists (a) or hands behind the back and gently lean backward. This is obviously easier to perform when sitting on a stool as a chair back can get in the way of the arms.

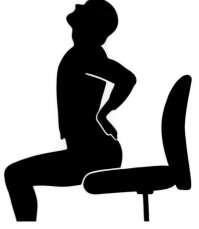

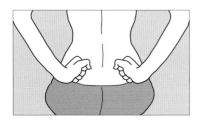

Exercise 8: Encouraging Lateral Flexion

This exercise is best performed sitting on a chair without armrests or on a stool. Keeping the arms close to the sides, lean to one side, thus producing lateral flexion of the spine. Repeat on the other side.

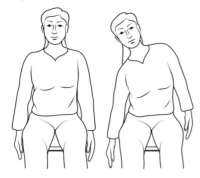

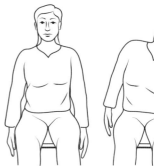

Exercise 9: Encouraging Rotation

When a subject has backache, attempting to perform seated rotation (a and b) is often painful. The images shown here are often used for stretching the lumbar spine. Encouraging rotation does not necessarily need to involve stretching; it can simply be just movement. An alternative is to use a swivel chair, like a five-wheeled office chair, and to use this to facilitate rotation. One method is to hold the edge of a desk and use the feet to rotate the chair, slowly turning the seat and pelvis and therefore the lumbar spine, or keeping the feet stationary and using the desk to push off from, gently rotating the chair first clockwise and then anticlockwise.

a
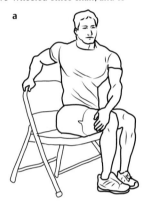

b
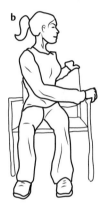

Tip 7: Encouraging Movement of the Lumbar Spine – Standing

In the standing position, the lumbar spine has to support the weight of the head, torso, and upper limbs. As we walk, the lumbar spine naturally changes shape, from flexion to extension in accordance with movements of the pelvis associated with each step. As we lift a foot from the ground, the spine also laterally flexes and rotates. Subjects who remain motionless for fear of pain risk a stiffening of the spine and ultimately this delays recovery.

The movements shown here are extremely subtle, relying on changes in weight-bearing or using a change in pelvic position to facilitate a change in lumbar posture. They are not designed to be performed in any order and clients are likely to prefer those that involve minimal movement to begin. Repeating each movement just two to five times is likely to be beneficial in increasing lumbar movement, reducing pain, and preventing stiffness.

Please read Tip 3 before using these techniques with your client.

Exercise 1: Side-to-Side Sway

Standing with feet hip-distance apart, body weight centralized, simply transfer weight onto the right foot (a), then back to center. From the center, transfer weight over to the left foot (b), and back to center again. Do not lift the feet from the floor. This swaying motion encourages lateral flexion of the spine.

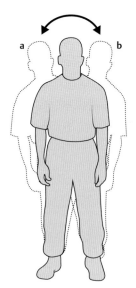

Exercise 2: Weight Transfer

With feet hip-distance apart (a) transfer weight onto the right foot but unlike in Exercise 1, this time lift your left foot a little from the floor (b). Return to center, with both feet on the floor (c); transfer weight to the left foot and gently lift the right foot from the floor (d). Return to center.

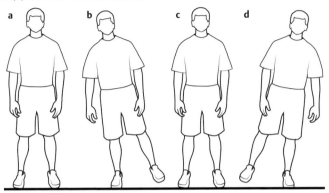

Exercise 3: Cross-Body Toe Taps

Using a railing, work surface, or table for support, for example, begin with the feet hip-distance apart (a). Transfer weight to the left leg and lift the right foot as in Exercise 2 (b); only this time, take the right leg across the body a little and tap the toe of the right foot on the ground (c). Return to the starting position (d). Repeat on the other side.

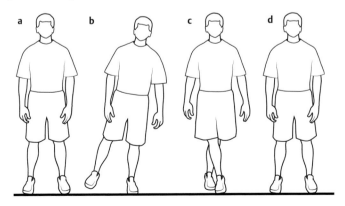

Exercise 4: Cross-Body Leg Swing

Once performing Exercise 3 is comfortable, try transferring weight onto one leg and instead of tapping the floor with the toe of the other leg, gently swing that leg back and forth. Repeat on the other side. This encourages gentle lateral flexion of the lumbar spine.

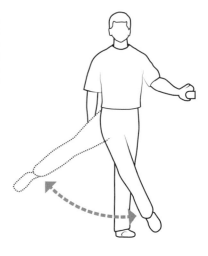

Exercise 5: Weight Transfer in Stance Phase

This is similar to Exercise 1; only instead of swaying side to side, the sway is forward and backward, trying to keep either the heel or the toe on the floor rather than lifting the foot entirely from the floor. The trick is to begin with one foot in front of the other (a) but keeping the legs slightly apart rather than trying to place them as one would on a tightrope. Lift the heel off the floor (b) and rock forward onto the front leg (c); take the weight off the front leg, lifting the toes (d), and transfer it back to the back leg, lowering the heel (e). Change legs and repeat in the other side.

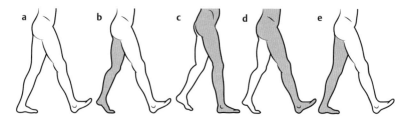

Exercise 6: Leg Swings

Once a client is comfortable with Exercise 5, they could use something to hold onto and practice gentle leg swinging forward and backward, first on one leg and then on the other leg. Leg swings produce flexion exterior of the lumbar spine.

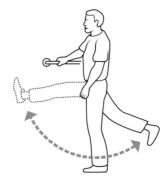

Exercise 7: Standing Hip Drops

For this exercise, your client will need something safe to stand on that is at least 2 in high. Standing with one foot off the step (a), lower that foot to the floor (b), dropping the hip to do this rather than pointing the toes. Raise the foot from the floor (c) and repeat with the other leg. This produces lateral flexion of the lumbar spine.

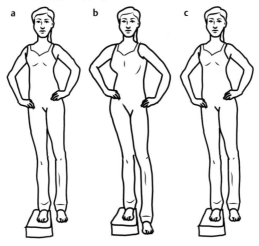

Tip 8: Increasing Activities of Daily Life for Clients with Back Pain

Activities of daily life or "ADLs," as termed by physical therapists, are everyday activities such as washing, dressing, cleaning, and shopping. Subjects with back pain find these extremely difficult to cope with, but research shows that people who return to normal ADLs as soon as possible fare far better than those who do not. This tip provides ideas for how a person with back pain can cope better with ADLs, and you may find it useful when treating clients who fall into this category.

Information has been compiled from a variety of sources including Bigos et al (1994), the Arthritis Research Council (2015, www.arthritisresearchuk.org), and Roland et al (2011), all of which are useful sources of further information.

There is no particular order to the information provided in this tip. It covers ADLs such as sleeping, washing, dressing, driving, shopping, household chores, and gardening. You could select from these categories those that which you feel are most appropriate, tailoring the information for each of your clients. With each activity, encourage your client to be as active as possible, gradually increasing the amount that they do in small increments. How quickly they progress is variable between individuals and may take days, weeks, or months; they should be discouraged from comparing themselves with other people they know who also have had back pain.

TIP: One of the best ways to learn about coping mechanisms for ADLS is to keep notes about what clients with back pain tell you themselves, what tricks they use to get through the day, how they pace themselves, and what devices they reply on.

Sleeping

For clients who report pain or stiffness in their low back in the morning, consider different ways of getting out of bed. For example:

A. Start in the side-lying position (a) and shuffle to the side of the bed; push up through

the elbow and arm, letting one leg to swing over the mattress (b). Use the arms to push the torso upright (c) until the client is able to sit on the edge of the bed (d).

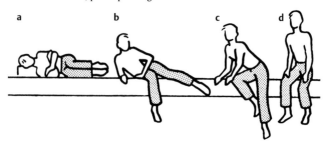

B. In the side-lying position (a), shuffle to the end of the bed. Turn onto knees and arms (b). Lower legs off the end of the bed, using the arms to push the torso upright (c).

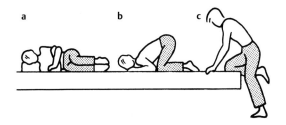

In the Bathroom

Back pain can be aggravated by reaching forward to turn the taps when in the bath, standing over a sink to brush teeth, or bending over to retrieve soap in the shower. Ways to overcome these issues include the following:

- Checking bath temperature before getting in and thus preventing adjustments.
- Using gels or soap on a rope when in the shower, which can be hooked to something at chest height.
- Kneeling rather than leaning over the bath to turn a tap or fit a plug.
- Using a selection of small towels because even lifting a large towel can be aggravating for subjects with acute back pain.
- Using microfiber mittens for drying instead of towels.
- Using a stool to rest the foot on for drying, reducing trunk flexion.
- Keeping a chair in the bathroom.
- Using a stool to raise the feet when using the toilet.

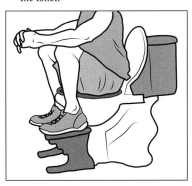

Dressing

Subjects with back pain report extreme difficulty with putting on socks, hosiery, and footwear. It can be helpful to use devices to assist such as long-handled grippers (a) or a shoehorn and to temporarily avoid wearing shoes that need lacing.

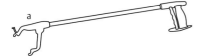

Other tips to help with dressing are to elevate the foot slightly onto a stool, step or stair, in order to put on shoes or socks. Take care however when standing to do this. Draw a foot stool close to a chair, remain sitting in the chair and put on socks or shoes that way. Or, remain lying in bed, supine if necessary, and partially dress before getting out of bed. Take care when slipping the arms into a jacket or coat, as this often involves slight rotation of the spine.

Driving

Usually, retention of a static posture for prolonged periods of time aggravates back pain and so many people with back pain find that driving is extremely uncomfortable and leaves them in pain for a while even after they have arrived at their destination. Useful advice includes the following:

- If you do need to drive, take regular breaks.
- Minimize the amount that you drive generally.
- Break up your journeys with stops. Get out of your car and move around.
- Have a small cushion handy to place behind your back to change the position of your back when driving.

- Consider adjusting the seat position.
- Use a headed pad behind your back for pain relief.

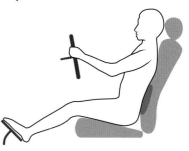

Shopping

- Consider shopping online and having groceries delivered to the door.
- Have a friend or family member available to help take in the delivery and put things away.
- If a supermarket visit is needed, take someone to help.

- Most supermarkets have staff to help, especially with loading items into a car. Ask for help.
- Avoid lifting. If lifting is essential, keep items close to the body. Take great care lifting things into and out of a car. Such positions put the spine under great load and often trigger an attack of back pain.

- Minimize the amount to be transported at any one time.
- If shopping locally, wherever possible use a wheeled trolley to transport items. The best kind for people with back pain is one that can be pushed in front of rather than wheeled behind the body as pulling a trolley involves rotation of the spine to one side, which can be aggravating.

- Avoid or minimize carrying. Keep items close to the body or split the load into two bags, one in each hand.
- When using a rucksack, be certain to carry it over both shoulders rather than one shoulder, so that the weight is centralized. Wear the rucksack high up on the back, not low down.

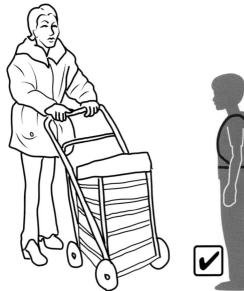

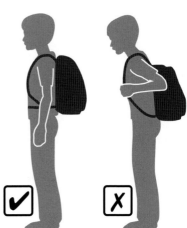

Laundry and Ironing

Everyone needs to do laundry and most people need to iron. These everyday activities can be hazardous for people with back pain and some clients report increasing anxiety when they see piles of washing or ironing piling up that needs to be done. Useful tips are as follows:

- Avoid retention of a static posture. Mix up stationary activities (such as ironing,

folding washing) with those that involve movement (such as light dusting).
- Avoid a twisting motion, as this too is harmful when back injuries occur. For example, putting washing into or out of a machine.
- Kneel or use a reaching device to help retrieve washing from a machine.

427

- Have someone else bring out the basket of washing prior to starting to iron.
- Ask a partner or family member to set up the ironing board.
- Use a lightweight iron.
- Adjust the height of the ironing board to prevent stooping.
- If sitting to iron is painful, consider standing (increasing the height of the ironing board accordingly).
- Avoid carrying multiple items of ironing at once in order to put them away.
- Use a wheeled basket to transport wet washing rather than lifting and carrying it. Or, instead of carrying wet washing to the line, take it piece by piece.
- It seems obvious, but instead of reaching up to hang washing, lower the wash-ing line where possible and hang the

washing that way before raising the line. Reaching up involves extension of the spine; this is extremely aggravating for some subjects with back pain.

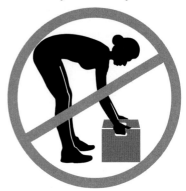

Cleaning

Cleaning usually involves performing a repetitive motion while bent over: floor brushing, floor washing, mopping, vacuum-ing, polishing, for example, all of which are potentially aggravating.

- Break up tasks, taking regular breaks to stretch the back.
- Use long-handled brushes and mops and try to remain upright when using these.
- When needing to plug in an appliance such as a vacuum cleaner, choose a me-dium height socket rather than stooping to use one close to the ground.

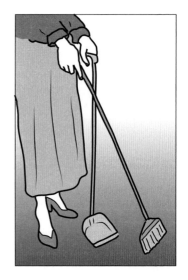

- Similarly, remain upright when vacuuming, moving slowly from one area to another rather than reaching forward and backward with a large motion.
- To clean a floor, rest on the knees and one hand, rather than flexing at the waist as this keeps the spine in a more neutral position. Work in a small area and then move to the next rather than using your arms in wide sweeping motions. Keep the cleaning equipment close and avoid twisting to wring out a cloth, for example.

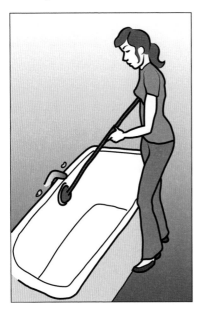

- When making beds, avoid lifting heavy mattresses to tuck in sheets. Consider using a lightweight foam mattress on top of a regular mattress as a temporary measure so that it is necessary to lift the corner of a lightweight mattress when fitting sheets. Injury often occurs when a subject shakes out a sheet or duvet, so take care with these activities.
- Collect household refuse in small bags to avoid having to lift a heavy refuse sack out of a dustbin.
- To use a sink to wash vegetables or dishes, place a folded towel between the edge of the sink and your stomach, and lean into this for support. If space allows, rest a foot on a stool and alternate feet frequently. Raise the height of the washing-up bowl by placing something beneath it.

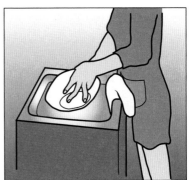

Cooking

- Avoid lifting heavy items such as large pans of water or a roast. Consider using a steamer where vegetables can be cooked together with less water, thereby making the pan lighter.

- Where possible, avoid stooping to use a low-level oven. If the oven is low, it might be helpful to use a slow cooker which does not need to be placed in an oven at all.

- Ask a family member to lift down plates from high shelves or cupboards and avoid carrying more than one plate at a time either when accessing these to serve food or when putting crockery away.
- Consider using a food trolley to transport food from the kitchen to where food will be eaten.

Work

There is strong evidence that a subject with back pain who stays off work for 1 to 2 years is unlikely to ever return to any form of work despite future treatment (Waddell and Burton 2001). A phased return to work may be appropriate and/or a modification in duties in the short term. Clients who have sedentary jobs may have as many difficulties as clients with physically demanding jobs. Most large organizations now have an occupational health department and it may be worth asking whether your client feels comfortable approaching occupational health practitioners for advice. Occupational health practitioners are best placed to liaise with the client and their employer and to make recommendations for adjustments to work such as a modification in hours, temporary use of equipment, or temporary adjustment of duties.

Exercise and Sport

Exercise is crucial to prevent weight gain, keep bones, muscles, and joints strong; retain cardiovascular fitness; and improve mood states. In most cases, it is very important for a client with back pain to keep moving, but obviously pain can limit participation in exercise and sport.

- Consider temporarily changing to a low-impact sport such as swimming or cycling.
- Swimming on the stomach can be aggravating, so consider water aerobics or pool walking/running and other pool-based exercises.
- Consider modifying existing sporting activity—play less frequently or for a reduced number of minutes.
- Attempt minimal amounts of walking and gradually build this up day by day.
- Consider gentle exercises such as tai chi.
- Temporarily avoid sports that involve retention of a static posture for prolonged periods of time, such as cycle racing.
- Temporarily avoid combat sports or sports that involve impact such as rugby.
- People with low back pain who are used to participation in sport can feel demoralized when unable to perform as they would normally. Keeping a sporting 'diary' and focusing on those activities that a subject *is* able to do can help a person feel more positive about their abilities and maintain morale.

Working at a Desk

We all need to sit at a desk from time to time, to pay bills, read, work on a computer or laptop.

- Take regular breaks.
- Make sure that when sitting, the chair is positioned correctly for the height of the desk.
- Consider using a seat wedge or lumbar support to alter the position of the back. Remove this from time to time so that the back rests in a different position.
- Consider using a chair with a seat that has a tilt function.

- Ensure you are sitting squarely to the desk, and not rotated to one side. Even very slight rotation can be detrimental to a subject with lumbar pain.
- Practice gentle mobility exercises whilst seated. These could be simple pelvic tilts anteriorly or posteriorly. Or, gentle rotation to one side. Note that rotation when performed in this manner is different to rotation that is present through a constant sitting posture. Moving into and out of a lumbar posture is likely to be beneficial whereas retention of a static lumbar posture is probably not.

Gardening

- Use long-handled gardening tools wherever possible.
- Avoid lifting or carrying. Split what has to be carried into smaller items wherever possible. For example, scoop out smaller amounts of compost rather than attempting to lift a large bag full.

- If possible, move things around a garden or patio on a wheeled trolley.
- Keep tools and equipment close by.
- Avoid the retention of a static posture for long periods of time.
- Kneel to weed rather than bending over.
- Take regular breaks to stretch the back.

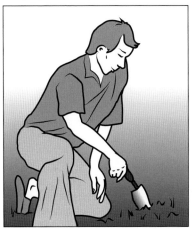 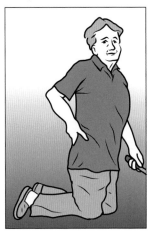

- Avoid carrying heavy bags of garden refuse.
- Avoid using a spade wherever possible as this is equivalent to lifting.
- Avoid reaching overhead to prune trees as this involves spine extension and can be aggravating. Small amounts of this kind of activity are good to intersperse with activities involving flexion, but neither should be performed for long periods of time without taking a break.
- Use a hose rather than a watering can and take care to avoid lifting a coiled hose, which can be heavy.
- Avoid reaching over anything. For example, leaning over a fence to prune a rose and leaning over a tray of seeds to retrieve a tool.
- Use lightweight tools where possible.
- When carrying, minimize the weight and keep it close to your body.
- Where possible, plant seeds in containers at waist height rather than stooping to the ground.
- Take care when lifting and hanging baskets.
- Even plastic tubs when filled with soil are heavy, so avoid moving these. If they need to be moved and must remain full, roll them on their bottom edge from one place to the other rather than attempting to lift them.

Tip 9: "Banana" Stretches for the Lumbar Spine

There are many ways to stretch the lateral flexors of the lumbar spine, yet some of the most simple and effective stretches are frequently overlooked. The stretches shown here are based on the movement of lateral flexion.

As you read through these examples, remember that the most effective stretches are those where the client can relax in the stretching position. When something is effortful, muscle tone increases. Therefore the more effort that is required to perform the stretch, the less effective it is likely to be. Stretches are effective when held for a minimum of 30 seconds and repeated daily (American College of Sports Medicine 2011).

The stretches illustrated here enable your client to select the degree of lengthening (stretch) they feel comfortable with, and can easily monitor their progress. If you are working with a client who has a stiff low back, or has suffered an injury or overworked the lateral flexors, you may wish to prescribe the most gentle of stretches, which is why, as with other tips in this section, you may wish to practice the stretches yourself to see how they feel and to use the table provided at the end of the tip to record your findings. Or you could use the table as a checklist for your client, giving them the option of using different stretches each week or progressing from the easier positions to those that are more challenging.

Let us begin with a really simple concept: if you move two ends of a muscle further apart, the muscle is required to lengthen. QL, a prime lateral flexor, has insertion points on the lower rib and the iliac crest (as well as the lumbar spine of course). Therefore, if the ribs and pelvis are moved apart, this muscle is lengthened.

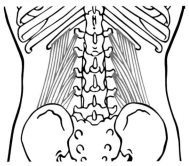

Moving the ribs away from the pelvis when the torso is kept on one plane produces a kind of banana shape to the body. As you go through this tip, ask yourself whether the ribs are moving away from the pelvis or whether the pelvis is moving away from the ribs, or both.

In this tip, you will find a whole range of stretches, which include stretches in the following positions: supine, squatting, prone, seated, kneeling, and standing.

Bananaring in Supine

Resting on the back, arms abducted, *slightly* flex the knees and hips. Keeping the torso still, use the feet to shuffle the lower limbs to one side, "bananaring" the body. Extend the knees and relax the hips so that both legs are touching, straightened, and to one side. The pelvis has been taken away from the ribs.

To increase the stretch, your client simply needs to elevate their arm on the convex side of the body. This elevates the ribs from the pelvis.

Start position   End position   Enhanced position

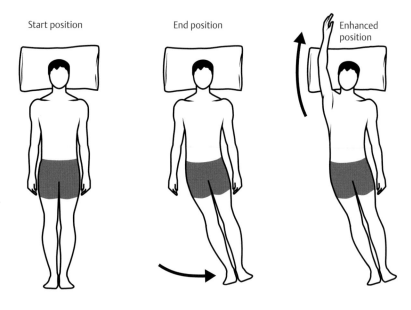

TIP: It is easier to use the legs to shuffle the lower part of the body to one side than it is to lift the torso and move that to one side.

Bananaring in Prone

This is slightly more difficult to achieve and instead of using the legs to take the hips away for the ribs, in this case it is easier for the client to rest on their elbows and "walk" their upper body to one side to create the banana shape, taking their ribs away from their pelvis.

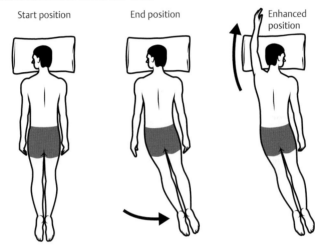

Start position   End position   Enhanced position

To increase the stretch, the client takes their pelvis away from their ribs, but in order to do this they would need to use their feet to shuffle their lower limbs to one side, and this is difficult in the prone position.

Bananaring on Four-Point Kneeling

Resting on their hands and knees, your client could "walk" their hands to one side, keeping the knees still.

Start position   End position

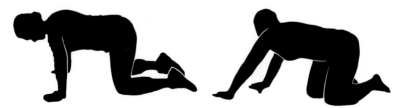

Bananaring in a Squat Position

A variation on this is to rest on the knees, sitting Japanese style, and then to "walk" the hands to one side.

End position (move either left or right)

Start position

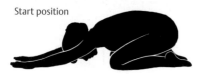

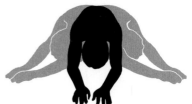

Side-Sitting Quadratus Lumborum Stretch

One of the simplest ways to stretch the lateral flexors is simply to push up from the side-lying position (taking the ribs away from the pelvis).

If you turn this image through 90 degrees so that the legs are vertical, you can see just how flexed the lateral spine is in this side-seated position. A modification is for your client to rest on their elbow rather than pushing up through a fully extended elbow.

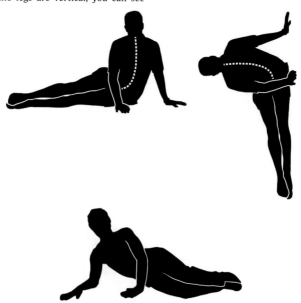

Side-Lying Quadratus Lumborum Stretch

Taking the pelvis away from the ribs requires the use of a bed or sturdy plinth.

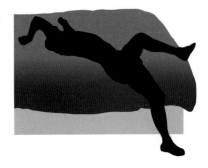

Standing Quadratus Lumborum Stretches

In the first of these stretches, the subject is using the wall for support and has taken their pelvis away from their ribs. In the sec-

ond, the client is enhancing the stretch by elevating their arm on the stretch side and "hanging" from a fencepost.

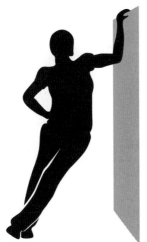

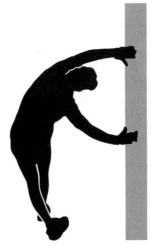

Notice that, taking the leg on the stretch side behind the body, in either stretch position, drops the hip and further enhances the stretch.

The following stretches are often portrayed as stretching QL, but are they effective? QL is a lateral flexor of the spine, so unless the subject is relaxed, the muscle holding them in the stretch position *is* QL, working iso-metrically (or even eccentrically) the very muscle that is purported to be being stretched.

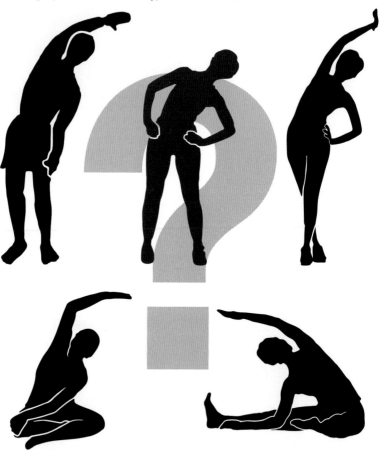

Stretch position	Comments
Bananaring in supine	
Bananaring in supine (enhanced)	
Bananaring in prone	
Bananaring in prone (enhanced)	

Stretch position	Comments
Bananaring in four-point kneeling 	
Bananaring in squat position 	
Side-sitting QL stretch 	
Side-sitting QL stretch (modified) 	

Abbreviation: QL, quadratus lumborum.

Stretch position	Comments
Side-lying QL stretch 	
Standing QL stretch (1) 	
Standing QL stretch (2) 	
?Other QL stretches 	

Abbreviation: QL, quadratus lumborum.

Tip 10: Rotatory Stretches for the Lumbar Spine

Tip 9 provided a selection of stretches for the lumbar spine based on lateral flexion. The stretches in this tip are all based on rotation. They include stretches in a variety of positions: sitting, supine, side lying, kneeling, and standing.

Just as for the lateral flexion stretches, the most effective stretches are those where the client can relax in the stretching position, and are most effective when held for a minimum of 30 seconds and repeated daily. The more effort that is required to attain the stretch, the less effective it is likely to be.

The stretching concept used here is the same as in Tip 9: if you take two ends of a muscle further apart, the muscle is required to lengthen. Tip 9 described how, if you move the insertion points of QL apart by laterally flexing the spine, you lengthen the muscle. The insertion points—the lower rib and the iliac crest—may also be moved apart in a different plane, by *rotating* either the torso or the pelvis or both. Rotation needs to be performed slowly and with care.

A table has again been provided at the end of this tip, which you could use to document your findings when practicing these stretches for yourself.

Simple Seated Rotation

It would seem logical that simply rotating the thorax in one direction stretches the lumbar spine by moving the ribs away from the pelvis (a). The disadvantage of this (and when using the modified version) is that it requires force to rotate the body and so may be of more benefit as a strengthening and mobility exercise than as a stretch for the lumbar spine.

Some people report feeling a greater stretch when they hook their arms over a broomstick (b) and rotate while seated (c).

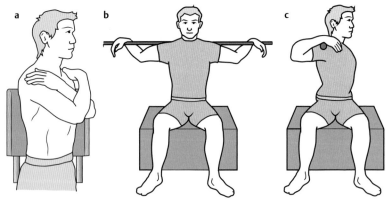

Seated Rotation Stretch

Feet firmly on the floor, your client attempts to rotate their thorax only. They may use the chair arms or the back of the chair to facilitate the stretch (a). Here the ribs are being rotated away from the pelvis. The stretch is enhanced further when attempting to look over one shoulder (b) (in the same direction as the stretch).

a

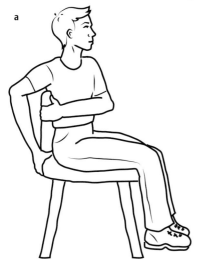

b

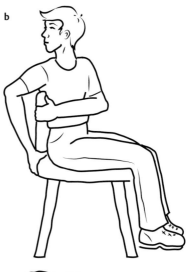

To enhance the stretch, your client could lean forward and then rotate, as demonstrated in this illustration. This enhances the stretch because it necessitates not only rotation but also flexion of the spine, and so stretches not only the lateral flexors, but also the lumbar extensor muscles.

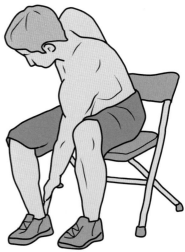

Simple Supine Hip Rotation

This is a relatively easy movement to perform, but even so can be uncomfortable for clients with reduced range of movement in the lumbar spine. Such clients should be encouraged to take their knees only as far as they feel comfortable, and not to worry if they cannot get both knees over to one side. In this stretch, the hips are rotated away from the ribs.

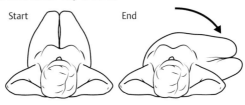

Start   End

Side-Lying Rotatory Stretch

Another way to take the ribs away from the pelvis is to begin resting in a side-lying position, hips and knees comfortably flexed, then to turn the torso supine, abducting one arm. This is a powerful stretch and can be uncomfortable for many clients, especially those with a reduced range of movement in the lumbar spine. In this stretch, the ribs are rotated away from the pelvis.

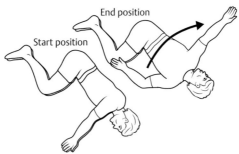

End position

Start position

TIP: Placing a small, soft ball or pillow beneath the knee reduces the degree of stretch, and extending the supporting leg also helps.

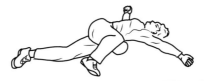

Standing Rotation Stretch

Another way to stretch the lumbar spine is in standing. With their back to a wall, your subject simply turns around as far as possible and tries to place their hands on the wall. This places rotatory force on the knees and ankles, which some clients could find uncomfortable. Conversely, as some of the force is taken up in the lower limb in this stretch, some clients may prefer this.

Kneeling Rotation Stretch

This stretch is actually designed to stretch the back of the shoulder, but as you can see from the illustration, a degree of supported lumbar rotation is required.

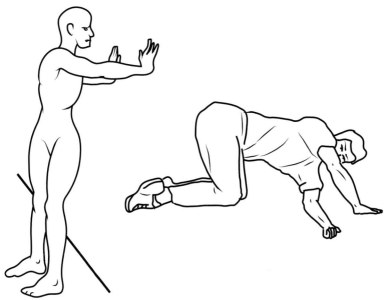

Stretch	Comments
Seated with no chair support	
Seated with broomstick	
Seated with back to chair	
Seated with side to chair	
Seated with flexion	
Simple hip rotationww	
Side-lying rotation stretch	
Standing rotation	
Kneeling rotation	

Tip 11: Rocking and Active Leg Swinging to Alleviate Low Back Pain

Rocking

Continuous passive motion while seated is an age-old remedy for back pain. Rocking chairs were once common in many homes but tend now to be seen as antiques rather than functional pieces of furniture. Rocking chairs produce a flexion/extension movement of the spine. A client could rest with the feet on the floor or elevated on a stool and gently rock themselves forward and backward using their legs rather than their back muscles.

There is no protocol for the use of a rocking chair for the treatment of low back pain. However, one study carried out in Finland (Niemelä et al 2011) with frail elderly subjects found that use of a home-based rocking chair exercise program lead to quantifiable improvements in physical performance. This study provides some illustrations of the kinds of exercises that were used, and while these may not be appropriate for clients with back pain, they could form a starting point for thinking about the use of a rocking chair as part of treatment.

In their study of 60 subjects with low back pain, van Deursen et al (1999) found that rotation of the seat base reduced pain. They note that the passive movements used in the study were of small amplitude and that it is not known why such movements reduced pain.

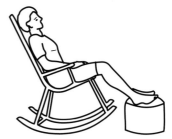

Swinging

Could the momentum generated by using a swing be used in a similar fashion to rocking chairs for the treatment of low back pain? Swinging requires knee extension and knee flexion, and contraction of abdominal muscles tends to occur on the knee extension "up" phase of swinging. Could this be beneficial to the alleviation of pain?

Alternatively, could the motion of simply swinging the legs when sitting on a static chair create enough minor movement in the spine to reduce symptoms? Swinging has been investigated as a form of physical pendulum (Post et al 2007). Neither static leg swinging nor whole-body swing-set swinging has been investigated for the use of back pain, but both utilize the same type of flexion/extension movement as when using a rocking chair. This suggests that they have potential as a rehabilitative tool.

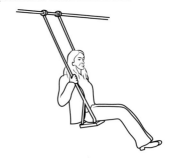

References

Abenhaim L, Rossignol M, Valat JP, et al. The role of activity in the therapeutic management of back pain: report of the International Paris Task Force on Back Pain. Spine 2000;25(Suppl 4):1S–33S

Adams MA, Hutton WC. The effect of posture on the lumbar spine. J Bone Joint Surg Br 1985;67(4):625–629

American Academy of Orthopaedic Surgeons. Joint Motion, Method of Measuring and Recording. Chicago, IL: American Academy of Orthopaedic Surgeons; 1965

American College of Sports Medicine. Quantity and quality of exercise for developing and maintaining cardiorespiratory, musculoskeletal, and neuromuscular fitness in apparently healthy adults: guidance for prescribing exercise. Med Sci Sports Exerc 2011;43(7):1334–1359

American Orthopaedic Association Web site. http://www.aoassn.org/

Arthritis Research UK. Keep Moving. [Leaflet], 2014.

Berry FB. Material on Thoracic Exercises Given to Patients at Thoracic Surgery Center, 160th General Hospital, European Theater of Operations, Surgery in World War II. Vol. I. Washington, DC: Medical Department, Office of the Surgeon General, Department of the Army; 1963

Beurskens AJ, de Vet HC, Köke AJ, et al. Efficacy of traction for nonspecific low back pain: 12 week and 6 month results of a randomized clinical trial. Spine 1997;22(23):2756–2762

Bigos S, Bowyer O, Braen G, et al. Acute Low Back Problems in Adults. Clinical Practice Guideline No. 14. AHCPR Publication No. 95-0642. Rockville, MD: Agency for Health Care Policy and Research, Public Health Service, US Department of Health and Human Services; 1994

Bockenhauer SE, Chen H., Julliard KN, Weedon J. Measuring thoracic excursion: reliability of the cloth tape measure technique. J Am Osteopath Assoc. 2007;107(5): 191–196

Braune W, Fischer O. Ueber den Schwerpunkt des Menschlichen Korpers mit Rücksicht auf die Ausrüstung des Deutschen Infanteristen. Abh. D. Kgl. Sächs. Ges. D. Wissensch. Math. Phys. Klasse 1889;26:562

British Orthopaedic Association Web site. http://www.boa.ac.uk/

Brunnstrom S. Clinical Kinesiology. Philadelphia, PA: F.A. Davis Company; 1972

Cloward RB. Cervical diskography: a contribution to the etiology and mechanism of neck, shoulder and arm pain. Ann Surg 1959;150(6):1052–1064

Davies C. The Trigger Point Therapy Workbook. Oakland, CA: New Harbinger; 2004

Duncan R. Integrated Myofascial Therapy Level 3 Workbook Notes & Technique Manual. Glasgow, UK: Myofascial Release; 2012

Dvořák J, Panjabi MM, Chang DG, Theiler R, Grob D. Functional radiographic diagnosis of the lumbar spine: flexion-extension and lateral bending. Spine 1991;16(5): 562–571

Earls J, Myers T. Fascial Release for Structural Balance. Berkley, CA: North Atlantic Books; 2010

Ezzo J, Haraldsson BG, Gross AR, et al. Massage for mechanical neck disorders: a systematic review. Spine (Philadelphia, PA, 1976) 2007;32:353–362

Fairbank JC, Couper J, Davies JB, O'Brien JP. The Oswestry low back pain disability questionnaire. Physiotherapy 1980;66:271–273

Fairbank JCT. William Adams and the Spine of Gideon Algernon Mantell. Ann R Coll Surg Engl 2004;86(5):349–352

Fallon S, Walsh M. Positional Release Technique: a valid technique for use by physical therapy practitioners. IPTAS Conference (2012), Wordpress.com

Fedorak C, Ashworth N, Marshall J, Paull H. Reliability of the visual assessment of cervical and lumbar lordosis: how good are we? Spine 2003;28(16):1857–1859

Franklin ME, Conner-Kerr T. An analysis of posture and back pain in the first and third trimesters of pregnancy. J Orthop Sports Phys Ther 1998;28(3)133–138

Fritz S. Sports & Exercise Massage. Philadelphia, PA: Elsevier; 2005

Furlan AD, Brosseau L, Imamura M, Irvin E. Massage for low-back pain: a systematic review within the framework of the Cochrane Collaboration Back Review Group. Spine 2002;27(17):1896–1910

Greene WB, Heckman JD, eds. The Clinical Measurement of Joint Motion. Rosemont, IL: American Academy of Orthopaedic Surgeons; 1994

Hertling D, Kessler RM. Management of Common Musculoskeletal Disorders. 3rd ed. Philadelphia, PA: Lippincott Williams & Wilkins; 1996

Hoving JL, O'Leary EF, Niere KR, Green S, Buchbinder R. Validity of the neck disability index, Northwick Park neck pain questionnaire, and problem elicitation technique for measuring disability associated with whiplash-associated disorders. Pain 2003;102(3):273–281

Iceton J, Harris WR. Treatment of winged scapula by pectoralis major transfer. J. Bone Joint Surg Br 1987;69(1):108–110

Iunes DH, Cecílio MBB, Dozza MA, Almeida PR. Quantitative photogrammetric analysis of the Klapp method for treating idiopathic scoliosis. Rev Bras Fisioter 2010;14(2): 133–140

Johnson J. Soft Tissue Release. Champaign, IL: Human Kinetics; 2009

Johnson J. Postural Assessment. Champaign, IL: Human Kinetics; 2012

Kapandji AI. The Physiology of the Joints. Vol. 3. The Spinal Column, Pelvic Girdle and Head. London: Churchill Livingstone; 2008

Kendall FP, McCreary EK, Provance PG. Muscles: Testing and function. 4th ed. Baltimore, MD: Lippincott Williams and Wilkins; 1993

Kopec JA, Esdaile JM, Abrahamowicz M, et al. The Quebec back pain disability scale: conceptualization and development. J Clin Epidemiol. 1996;49(2):151–161

Krause M, Refshauge KM, Dessen M., Boland R. Lumbar spine traction: evaluation of effects and recommended application for treatment. Man Ther 2000;5(2):72–81

Leak AM, Cooper J, Dyer S, Williams KA, Turner-Stokes L, Frank AO. The Northwick Park Neck Pain Questionnaire, devised to measure neck pain and disability. Br J Rheumatol 1994;33:469–474

Lee LJ. Is it possible to be too stable? Ortho Div Rev 2006;(Nov/Dec):19–23

Lee LJ. Is it time for a closer look at the thorax? In Touch 2008; (1):13–16

Lemos TV, Albino AC, Matheus JP, Barbosa Ade M. The effect of kinesio taping in forward bending of the lumbar spine. J Phys Ther Sci. 2014;26(9):1371–1375

Lord MJ, Small JM, Dinsay JM, Watkins RG. Lumbar lordosis: effects of sitting and standing. Spine 1997;22(21): 2571–2574

Maigne R. Origine dorso-lombaire de certaines lombalgies basses. Rôle des articulations interapophysaires et des branches postérieures des nerfs rachidiens. Rev Rhum 1974;41(12):781–789

Maitland J. Spinal Manipulation Made Simple: A Manual of Soft Tissue Techniques. Berkeley, CA: North Atlantic Books; 2001

Malmivaara A, Häkkinen U, Aro T, et al. The treatment of acute low back pain—bed rest, exercises, or ordinary activity? N Engl J Med. 1995; 332(6):351–355

Manheim CJ, Lavett DK. The Myofascial Release Manual. Thorofare, NJ: Slack Incorporated; 1989

Martin RM, Fish DE. Scapular winging: anatomical review, diagnosis, and treatments. Curr Rev Musculoskelet Med 2008;1(1): 1–11

McKenzie AM, Taylor NF. Can physiotherapists locate lumbar spinal levels by palpation? Physiother 1997;83(5):235–239

McPartland JM, Brodeur RR, Hallgren RC. Chronic neck pain, standing balance, and suboccipital muscle atrophy–a pilot study. J Manipulative Physiol Ther 1997;20(1): 24–29

Mears R. Bushcraft Survival, Series 1 [DVD], BBC; 1996

Min SH, Chang S-H, Jeon SK, Yoon SZ, Park J-Y, Shin HW. Posterior auricular pain caused by the trigger points in the sternocleidomastoid muscle aggravated by psychological factors—a case report. Korean J Anesthesiol 2010; 59:S229–S232

Moll JMH, Wright V. Normal range of spinal mobility. Ann Rheum Dis 1971;30:3 81–386

Moll JMH, Wright V. Measurement of spinal movement. In: Jayson M., ed. The Lumbar Spine and Back Pain. New York: Grune & Stratton; 1981:93–112

Moseley GL. Impaired trunk muscle function in patients with sub-acute neck pain: etiologic in the subsequent development of low-back pain. Man Ther. 2004;9:157–163

Mulligan BR. Manual Therapy: NAGS, SNAGS, MWMS, etc. Wellington, New Zealand: Plane View Services Ltd; 2010

Nachemson A, Elfström G. Intravital dynamic pressure measurements in lumbar discs: a study of common movements, maneuvers and exercises. Scand J Rehabil Med 1970;2(Suppl 1):1–40

Niemelä K, Väänänen I, Leinonen R, Laukkanen P. Benefits of home-based rocking-chair exercise for physical performance in community-dwelling elderly women: a randomized controlled trial—a pilot study. Aging Clin Exp Res 2011;23(4):279–287

Nissen H. Practical Massage and Corrective Exercises. Philadelphia, PA: F.A. Davis Company; 1905

Norkin CC, White DC. Measurement of Joint Motion: A Guide to Goniometry. Philadelphia, PA: F.A. Davis Company; 1985

Ohashi W. Do-It-Yourself Shiatsu. London: Unwin Paperbacks; 1977

Paulin E, Brunetto AF, Carvalho CRF. Effects of a physical exercise program designed to increase thoracic expansion in chronic obstructive pulmonary disease patients. J Pneumologia 2003;29(5):287–294

Pavelka K. Rotations - messung der Wirbelsaule. Z Rheumaforsch 1970;29:366–370

Pearcy M, Portek I, Shepherd J. Three-dimensional x-ray analysis of normal movement in the lumbar spine. Spine 1984a;9(3):294–297

Pearcy MJ, Tibrewal SB. Axial rotation and lateral bending in the normal lumbar spine measured by three-dimensional radiography. Spine 1984b;9(6):582–587

Petias P, Grivas TB, Kaspiris A, Aggouris C, Evangelos D. Review of the trunk surface metrics used as scoliosis and other deformities evaluation indices, Scoliosis 2010;5:12

Post AA, de Groot G, Daffertshofer A, Beek PJ. Pumping a playground swing. Motor Control 2007;11(2):136–50

Proctor D, Dupuis P, Cassidy JD. Thoracolumbar syndrome as a cause of low back pain: a report of two cases. J Can Chiropr Assoc 1985;29(2):71–73

Quebec Back Pain Disability Scale. http://www.backpainscale.ca/. Accessed July 19, 2015

Roland M, Waddell G, Moffett JK, Burton K, Main C. The Back Book: The Best Way to Deal with Back Pain; Get Back Active. Norwich, UK: Stationary Office (STO); 2011

Rose J. Upper back: osteopathic lesions in the thoracic spine. http://www.holistic-doc-pain support.com/ thoracic-spine.html. 2008

Sahrmann SA. Does postural assessment contribute to patient care? J Orthop Sports Phys Ther 2002;32(8):376–379

Sherman KJ, Cherkin DC, Hawkes RJ, Miglioretti DL, Deyo RA. Randomized trial of therapeutic massage for chronic neck pain. Clin J Pain, 2009;25:233–238

Shin S, Yoon DM, York KB. Identification of the correct cervical level by palpation of spinous processes. Anesth. Analog 2011;112(5):1232–1235

Solberg G. Postural Disorders and Musculoskeletal Dysfunction: Diagnosis, Prevention and Treatment. Edinburgh, UK: Churchill Livingstone; 2008

Struyf F, Nijs J, De Coninck K, Giunta M, Mottram S, Meesen R. Clinical assessment of scapula positioning in musicians: an intertester reliability study. J Athl Train 2009;44(5):519–526

van Deursen, LL, Patijn J, Durinck JR, Brouwer R, van Erven-Sommers JR, Vortman BJ. Sitting and low back pain: the positive effect of rotatory dynamic stimuli during prolonged sitting. Eur Spine J 1999;8(3):187–193

Vanti C, Bertozzi L, Gardenghi I, Turoni F, Guccioni AA, PIllastrini P. Effect of taping on spinal pain and disability: systematic review and meta-analysis of randomized trials. Phys Ther 2015;95(4):493–506

Verbunt JA, Seelen HA, Vlaeyen JW, et al. Disuse and deconditioning in chronic low back pain: concepts and hypotheses on contributing mechanisms. Eur J Pain 2003;7(1):9–21

Vernon H, Mior S. The Neck Disability Index: a study of reliability and validity. J Manipulative Physiol Ther 1991;14:409–415

Waddell G, Burton AK. Occupational health guidelines for the management of low back pain at work: evidence review. Occup Med 2001;51(2):124–135

Wall P. Pain: The Science of Suffering. London: Weidenfeld & Nicolson; 1999

Watson AHD, William C, James BV. Activity patterns in latissimus dorsi and sternocleidomastoid in classical singers. J Voice 2012;26(3):e95–e105

Yin P, Gao N, Wu J, Litscher G, Xu S. Adverse events of massage therapy in pain-related conditions: a systematic review. Evid Based Complement Alternat Med 2014;1–11

Index

Page numbers in *italics* refer to illustrations